Pacing Options in the Adult Patient with Congenital Heart Disease

This book is dedicated to my family:
To my beloved wife, Evelynne, who has supported me through three books, numerous book chapters and hundreds of manuscripts. At times, I have felt that our marriage was a kinky ménage à trois; Evelynne, Harry and the computer.

To my children, Jonathan, Dean and Natalie, their spouses Tamara and Marty and my grandchildren, Jasmin, Olivia and Brodie.

Thank you all for providing so much joy and happiness to my life.

Harry G Mond

This book is dedicated to my family for all the support and encouragement given to me over many years, over many obstacles. I thank my mentors and friends in the fields of congenital heart cardiology and pacemaker design technologies, especially Paul Gillette, MD and Kenneth Stokes, BCh. I also thank Charles Mullins, MD, for his instructive schematic drawings of congenital heart anatomy.

My sincerest appreciation to all.

Peter P Karpawich

Pacing Options in the Adult Patient with Congenital Heart Disease

Harry G Mond, MBBS, MD, FRACP, FCSANZ, FHRS, FACC, DDU

Associate Professor, Department of Medicine, University of Melbourne
Honorary Associate Professor, Department of Epidemiology and Preventive Medicine,
Nursing and Health Sciences, Monash University, Melbourne
Specialist Physician, Department of Cardiology
The Royal Melbourne Hospital, Victoria, Australia

Peter P Karpawich, MD, FAAP, FACC

Professor, Department of Pediatrics, Wayne State University School of Medicine
Director, Cardiac Electrophysiology and Pacemaker Services
Children's Hospital of Michigan, Detroit, Michigan, USA

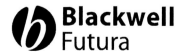
Blackwell
Futura

© 2007 Harry G. Mond, Peter P. Karpawich
Published by Blackwell Publishing
Blackwell Futura is an imprint of Blackwell Publishing

Blackwell Publishing, Inc., 350 Main Street, Malden, Massachusetts 02148-5020, USA
Blackwell Publishing Ltd, 9600 Garsington Road, Oxford OX4 2DQ, UK
Blackwell Science Asia Pty Ltd, 550 Swanston Street, Carlton, Victoria 3053, Australia.

First published 2007

1   2007

ISBN-13: 978-1-4051-5569-4
ISBN-10: 1-4051-5569-8

Library of Congress Cataloging-in-Publication Data
Mond, Harry G.
    Pacing options in the adult patient with congenital heart disease /
Harry G. Mond, Peter P. Karpawich.
    p. ; cm.
    Includes bibliographical references and index.
    ISBN-13: 978-1-4051-5569-4 (alk. paper)
    ISBN-10: 1-4051-5569-8 (alk. paper)
    1. Congenital heart disease. I. Karpawich, Peter P. II. Title.
    [DNLM: 1. Heart Defects, Congenital–surgery. 2. Adult. 3. Cardiac Pacing,
Artificial–methods. 4. Defibrillators, Implantable.
    WG 220 M741p 2007]
    RC687.M66 2007
    616.1'2043–dc22
                                                                2006018505

A catalogue record for this title is available from the British Library.

Acquisitions: Gina Almond
Development: Beckie Brand
Set in 10/13 Palatino by Newgen Imaging Systems (P) Ltd., Chennai, India
Printed and bound in Singapore by COS Printers Pte Ltd.

For further information on Blackwell Publishing, visit our website:
www.blackwellcardiology.com

The publisher's policy is to use permanent paper from mills that operate a sustainable
forestry policy, and which has been manufactured from pulp processed using acid-free and
elementary chlorine-free practices. Furthermore, the publisher ensures that the text paper
and cover board used have met acceptable environmental accreditation standards.

Contents

Introduction

As a consequence of an increasing understanding of congenital heart disease, there have been improvements in surgical correction or palliation, and many children born with serious or complicated structural cardiac abnormalities are now living up to adulthood. Because of their anatomical malformation or scarring from previous therapeutic interventions, serious bradyarrhythmias and tachyarrhythmias are now being frequently encountered. As these patients are now being managed by internal medicine-trained cardiologists, they are generally referred to an adult electrophysiology or pacemaker center for implantation of a pacemaker or Implantable cardioverter-defibrillator (ICD).

Thus, it is likely that all pacemaker or ICD implanters will, on occasion, encounter a patient with adult congenital heart disease. It, therefore behooves the implanter to have a general understanding of the surgical options available. The operator will need to determine if the transvenous approach is feasible, what problems may be encountered during the procedure and most importantly, how to negotiate the leads to the most appropriate intracardiac positions. On other occasions, the operator may be unaware of the congenital abnormality, but certain radiographic clues will be helpful in rapidly understanding the anatomy, thus minimizing the operative and fluoroscopy times.

This text will attempt to classify the different groups of patients with adult congenital heart disease, summarize the difficulties that may be encountered with the transvenous approach to lead placement and make recommendations as to the choice of hardware and the best surgical approach.

The authors of this text are both familiar with these scenarios, but in different arenas. Harry Mond is an adult cardiologist, who has been implanting cardiac pacemakers for over 36 years. His first experience with adult congenital heart disease was in 1971 at a time when pacing leads had no lumen for a stylet and instead required a large bore catheter in order to pass the floppy lead to the right ventricle. The case in question was a left superior vena cava and after many hours of lead manipulation, successful unipolar ventricular pacing was achieved, but via the middle cardiac vein. The case is illustrated in Figure 60. In that era, there were no experienced implanters to supervise and mentor, nor were the tools and implantable hardware user friendly. A left superior vena cava was essentially an unsuspected autopsy oddity with little or no clinical significance. It was not surprising, therefore, that most adult cardiologists had barely heard of and most certainly had no experience with this congenital abnormality. From that first potential fiasco, the next 35 years of pacemaker surgery presented the complete spectrum of congenital cardiac abnormalities of which the fluoroscopic, chest radiographic and other graphic teaching mementoes have been carefully collected and presented in this text.

In contrast, Peter Karpawich is a pediatric cardiologist with extensive experience in pacemaker implantation and design in patients with congenital heart disease. During his pediatric cardiology training in the late 1970s, cardiac electrophysiology and pacemaker application technologies in children with congenital heart defects were just emerging as sub-specialized fields of study. Over the past 25 years, those fields have attained new significance as young children with congenital heart disease are now attaining adulthood and will continue to require individuals with expertise in congenital heart anatomy and physiology. Associated with this new field of study, Dr Karpawich has worked closely with the pacing industry in the design and application of more efficient lead and generator technologies to both facilitate implant and extend battery longevity with wide applications to this emerging patient group.

Because there is very little written on the topic of pacemaker and ICD implantation in adult congenital heart disease, the authors have joined together to create such a text utilizing their individual expertise. This book outlines the principles of dealing with such patients including the preferences of techniques and the hardware available. The text is divided into two sections:

Part I describes the "tricks of the trade." Although prepared primarily for adult patients with congenital heart disease, the principles espoused are equally relevant for most patients who require cardiac pacing. The first section deals with preparing for the implant, problems that may be encountered on the way and tricks that are available for the seemingly impossible implant.

Part II classifies adult congenital heart disease patients into those patients who have and those who have not had previous corrective or palliative cardiac surgery. This part is further subdivided according to the level of challenge the operator will face.

As many of the implanters will be unsure of the anatomy, particularly in relation to the pathways to the venous atrium and ventricle, there is liberal use of simple line illustrations. Terminology common to the pediatric cardiologist, but possibly unfamiliar to the adult implanter is explained in simple "adult" language.

PART 1

Tricks of the trade

To many implanters, the adult patient with congenital heart disease conjures up a frightening surgical scenario. Although the implanting physician may be familiar during the training years with the array of congenital defects, such familiarity becomes clouded and obscure as years progress. Irrespective of how familiar the cardiac defect is to the implanting physician, once consideration is given as to how a lead will progress through the venous channels to the heart and then be positioned in the atrium or ventricle, a degree of uncertainty and fear emerges. In addition, it must be remembered, that a "repaired" congenital heart defect may not be synonymous with a "normal" heart. The post-operative anatomy may introduce many technical challenges to the implanting physician, attempting a pacemaker or ICD implant.

Consequently, as any pediatric cardiologist recognizes, a pacemaker or ICD implantation in a child with congenital heart disease requires special consideration and the procedure cannot be regarded as routine. Such special consideration must obviously be extrapolated to the adult scenario, where the implanting physician is usually less familiar with the anatomy than the pediatric counterpart. It is the objective of this part to outline the various principles required, when preparing for an implant in an adult patient with congenital heart disease. Most implanters will be familiar with a number of these general principles in regard to routine implants. However, they become more important in hearts with congenital abnormalities or obstructive post-operative scarring and are worth reviewing in detail. The authors will discuss the management of these potential problems and advise on the array of hardware options available. It is hoped that these principles will also be helpful for all implants.

CHAPTER 1

Know the anatomy

Prior to pacemaker or ICD implantation, a full understanding of the cardiovascular anatomy of the adult with congenital heart disease is critical.

• Can a lead be placed in a venous atrium or ventricle which leads to the pulmonary circulation?

• What are the fluoroscopic appearances and do they differ from the normal?

• Are the vascular pathways to the heart intact and otherwise normal?

Throughout this text, simple line diagrams will be used to explain the congenital abnormalities of the heart. These diagrams will in turn be compared to fluoroscopic or chest radiographic images with implanted leads. This will enable the reader to quickly grasp the anatomical variations to be found at surgery. The schematic diagram of a normal heart is shown in Figure 1.1.

In many instances, a pre-operative transthoracic or transesophageal echocardiogram, venogram, computerized tomographic scan or magnetic resonance imaging study will be necessary to define structures. A review of a relevant cardiac catheterization or surgical report may reveal an absent or obstructed superior vena cava or an innominate vein. The coronary sinus may not drain directly into the right atrium and with an Ebstein's anomaly of the tricuspid valve, the surgeon, in order to prevent heart block, may position the prosthetic tricuspid valve, so that the coronary sinus lies on the ventricular side of the valve. A few minutes spent, carefully checking the anatomy may save hours of anguish at the time of device implant.

Another potential troublesome abnormality in a patient is an interrupted inferior vena cava. In this situation, the right atrium receives only hepatic venous blood from below. The infrahepatic portion of the inferior vena cava is absent or rudimentary. Blood flow from the inferior vena cava to right atrium must reroute to a right or left superior vena cava via a right or

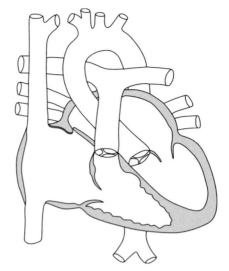

Figure 1.1 Schematic of a normal heart.

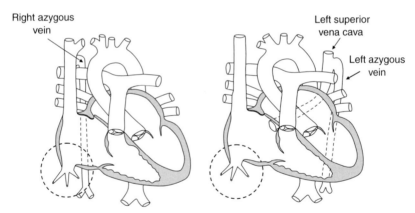

Right azygous vein

Left superior vena cava

Left azygous vein

Figure 1.2 Schematic appearance of variations of systemic venous return associated with interruption of the inferior vena cava. *Left:* A right azygous vein drains blood from the lower trunk into the superior vena cava. *Right:* A left azygous (hemiazygous) vein drains blood from the lower trunk into a left superior vena cava and from there into the right atrium via the coronary sinus.

left-sided azygous vein (Figure 1.2). Knowledge of this anatomical variant is important for anyone contemplating preoperative temporary pacing from a femoral vein site, lead extraction or any cardiac catheterization procedure. It will also be important to recognise if the superior pacing lead follows a strange course away from a right or left superior vena cava.

To the adult pacemaker and ICD implanter, many of the complex and even simple congenital cardiac anatomical abnormalities become very confusing; when transvenous leads need to be positioned in the atrium of ventricle. Many implanters have never considered such scenarios or have not encountered them for many years and consequently cannot envisage the anatomical pathways. A patient with congenital atrioventricular block or long QT interval without other anatomical abnormalities is considered a normal implant. However, congenitally corrected L-transposition of the great vessels, dextrocardia or maybe Ebstein's anomaly, although technically similar to the normal implant, may present implant challenges which can be easily overcome by a review of the anatomy. In other situations, such as surgically corrected D-transposition of the great vessels or persistent left superior vena cava, the anatomical challenges can be formidable to the uninitiated.

CHAPTER 2

Transvenous pacemaker implantation

A young patient with congenital heart disease, even with previous surgical scars, deserves the finest possible cosmetic result from a pacemaker or ICD implantation. The subclavicular incision remains the best long-term option if new leads are required in the future using the same incision. However, an alternative approach at the antero-axillary fold will allow access to the subclavian vein, whilst at the same time hiding the incision in the axilla [1]. This approach, commonly limited to females, requires a venogram to demonstrate the vein and a second incision under the breast for pulse generator placement. However, it is important to remember that a previous open thoracotomy associated with congenital heart surgery as a child may result in chest wall deformities and vascular distortion later in life which can complicate standard vascular access for lead insertion.

The subclavicular approach allows rapid access by the cutdown technique to the cephalic vein, avoiding the use of a subclavian puncture with all its recognized complications [2, 3]. Implanters familiar with the technique of cephalic vein isolation and cannulation can rapidly implant one or more leads, even in a small vein. In order to achieve this, many implanting physicians now use introducers in order to pass the leads into the proximal veins [4]. These introducers are best inserted using a very floppy flexible tip guide wire which is passed along the vein to the heart (0.89 mm/0.035″ flexible tip Radifocus®Glidewire® – Terumo Corporation, Tokyo, Japan) (Figure 2.1). Short 80cm wires are available for this purpose. The wire has a nitinol core, which is composed of a super-elastic nickel titanium alloy. It is then covered with radio-opaque polyurethane and coated with a hydrophilic polymer.

Once the cephalic vein is isolated and cleaned, the distal end is ligated and the proximal end secured using absorbable suture. A small transverse incision is made with fine or iris scissors and the intima observed or free bleeding is seen coming from the incision. The funnel introducer supplied with the guide wire is inserted into the vein and, provided the passageway

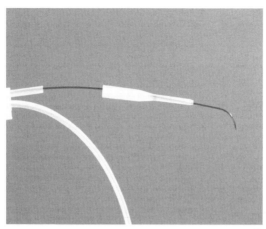

Figure 2.1 Terumo flexible tip, 0.89 mm (0.035″), Radifocus® Glidewire® (reproduced with permission from Terumo Corporation, Japan). See text for details.

is not obstructed, blood wells up in the funnel. The guide wire is then introduced and passed under fluoroscopic vision to the right heart (Figure 2.2). A standard introducer is passed over it (Figure 2.3). For a dual chamber implant, where the leads require 7F introducers, it is easier to use a 9F introducer, retaining the guide wire, which is secured to the surgical drape. The first lead is then passed into the introducer running parallel to the retained guide wire (Figure 2.3). Once the ventricular lead is positioned, a 7F introducer is passed over the guide wire and the atrial lead inserted and positioned (Figure 2.4).

On occasion, the cephalic vein may break during lead insertion. If the two leads cause a very tight fit in the vein, it may, as a consequence, invaginate the vein into the subclavian vein. The torn cephalic vein then produces a choking collar around the leads preventing positioning of the atrial lead (Figure 2.5). In this situation, the atrial lead should be carefully removed.

When the cephalic vein is too small or cannulation unsuccessful, the use of the retro-pectoral veins immediately deep to the clavicular head of the pectoralis major muscle should be considered [5, 6]. This is simply an extension of the cephalic vein cutdown and is familiar to most implanters who use the cephalic vein. These veins may be of a similar size to the cephalic vein and thus able to take two leads. Although the dissection is a little more extensive and the muscle must be gently retracted, a suitable vein can often be found. Similarly, anterior pectoral veins can be used but may require more extensive and painful dissection [7].

Prior to the introduction of the subclavian puncture, the external jugular vein was a common venous entry site for transvenous lead insertion. The

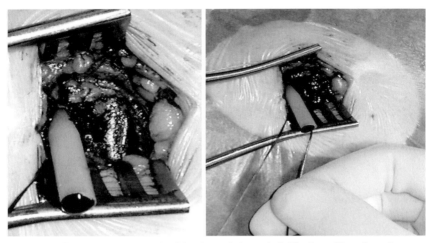

Figure 2.2 Cephalic vein retained guide wire technique. *Left:* The funnel introducer is inserted into the cephalic vein. Blood wells back. *Right:* The guide wire is inserted into the funnel.

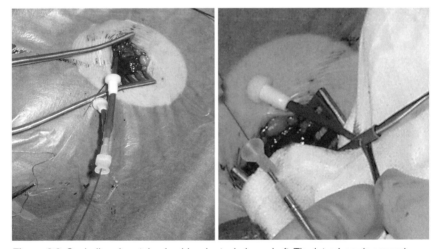

Figure 2.3 Cephalic vein retained guide wire technique. *Left:* The introducer is passed along the guide wire into the cephalic vein. *Right:* The dilator of the introducer is removed leaving the guide wire. The lead is then inserted parallel to the guide wire.

technique, however, had many disadvantages. Cannulation of the vein was difficult particularly in right heart failure and high venous pressures. The lead had to be manipulated under the clavicle to the heart and then once positioned and secured, a second subclavicular incision made and the lead brought down anterior and thus superficial to the clavicle. The lead, in this position in the neck was unsightly, uncomfortable and prone to erosion

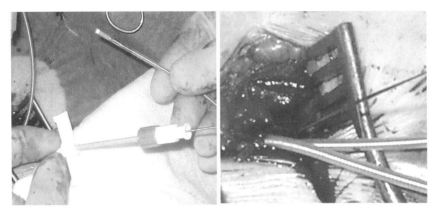

Figure 2.4 Cephalic vein retained guide wire technique. *Left:* A second introducer is inserted over the retained guide wire. *Right:* The second lead is inserted into the cephalic vein.

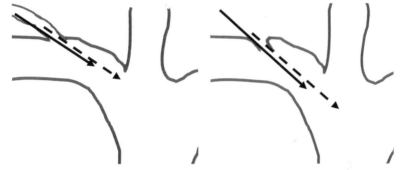

Figure 2.5 Schematic of the cephalic vein retained guide wire technique. *Left:* Two leads are passed along an intact cephalic vein. *Right:* The cephalic vein is torn with pushing of the second lead into the subclavian vein. The vein is then invaginated into the subclavian vein enclosing the two leads in a tight collar.

or fracture. Tunneling the lead deep to the clavicle has been reported [8]. There is no place for external jugular lead implantation today. Similarly, the internal jugular approach has many of the same complications including damage to the vagus nerve.

When the cephalic vein is not available, Seldinger puncture and cannulation of the axillary [9, 10] or subclavian veins should be considered. The implantation techniques have been widely reported and are standard procedures [11, 12]. Despite the benefits of the cutdown techniques and axillary puncture, the subclavian puncture technique remains the major venous access site for pacemaker and ICD implantation.

When the superior vena caval approach to the right heart is inaccessible, the decision is usually made to use the epicardial approach. However, there are a number of approaches using the inferior vena. The ilio-femoral route has been recommended as a venous access site for both single and dual chamber permanent pacemakers. The original procedure was actually performed by venous cutdown onto the saphenous vein as it entered the femoral vein and lead insertion was performed in a manner similar to a cephalic cutdown approach [13].

Later the iliac or femoral veins were used and lead insertion achieved by Seldinger puncture and introducer. The actual vein used depends on whether the puncture is above or below the inguinal ligament. The more common approach uses the iliac vein particularly if the pulse generator is to be implanted in the abdomen [14, 15]. In this situation the lead must take a sharp almost 360° turn from its entry into the vein to its passage up the anterior abdominal wall. With the vigorous activity of the leg relative to the immobile iliac vein, the lead is subject to marked stresses with the fulcrum being at the venous entry site. Thus the lead may be subject to fracture. Two incisions are required with one over the puncture site and the other in the abdominal wall although a single incision with a low pulse generator site has been reported [16].

The transfemoral approach is lower and in this situation the pulse generator or ICD may be positioned in the thigh [17, 18]. It must be remembered that for patients with congenital heart disease, an interrupted inferior vena cava needs to be excluded (Figure 1.2).

On rare occasions, other methods of venous access to the inferior vena cava have been reported in patients with complex congenital heart disease and no access to the heart from above. These include transhepatic cannulation [19] and an extra-peritoneal approach directly to the inferior vena cava [20]. For all these techniques, active fixation leads are obviously recommended in both the atrium and ventricle, because of the abnormal approaches to the heart from below.

CHAPTER 3

The pulse generator or ICD pocket

Another important consideration for the implanter is where to bury the pulse generator or ICD. In the chest, should the hardware lie on (prepectoral) or deep (subpectoral) to the pectoralis major muscle? The major concern with the prepectoral subcutaneous implant is the prominence of the implanted hardware including the extra vascular leads. This is particularly so if the pocket is within the adipose tissue rather than directly on the pectoral major fascia (Figure 3.1). As might be anticipated, the young active adolescent or adult may be more prone to trauma to the pulse generator or ICD site than a more sedentary older patient, resulting in skin necrosis and pulse generator, ICD or lead erosion (Figure 3.2).

In the years following pacemaker and ICD implantation, there is a gradual loss of the covering adipose tissue, particularly at the edges and

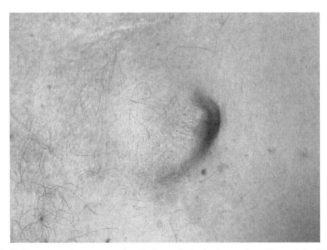

Figure 3.1 Pulse generator pre-erosion in the subclavicular region. The original implant was prepectoral. Following pulse generator replacement, the different shape pulse generator resulted in stresses at the lateral edge and pre-erosion.

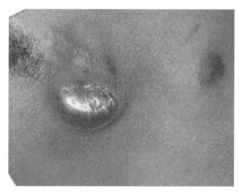

Figure 3.2 Pulse generator erosion in a newly implanted pulse generator. The patient started lifting weights one week post-implant and was unaware that the erosion was a problem.

corners of the implanted hardware. The resorption of the subcutaneous tissues is accelerated following pulse generator or ICD replacement and if the unit has a different shape, the overlying skin often becomes thin, painful and reddened, generally over the lateral edge. In such situations, the hardware will need repositioning and preferably buried deep to the pectoralis major muscle.

Another issue with the prepectoral implant, particularly in the young inquisitive adult, is the pacemaker and ICD twiddler's syndrome. This results from repeated twisting of the pulse generator or ICD in the subcutaneous pocket with eventual lead retraction, lead fracture and device malfunction (Figures 3.3, 3.4) [21–30].

For all these reasons, a number of implanters have recommended a subpectoral pocket [1, 31]. In this position, the cosmetic result is usually excellent. A subpectoral implant may better protect the active recipient from trauma, potential erosion and the twiddler's syndrome. Despite this, twiddling has been reported in the subpectoral pocket [32]. As a routine all pacemaker and ICD patients and, in particular, the young recipient, should be educated in the care of the pacemaker pocket and wound.

Despite this, there remains a controversy regarding the subpectoral implant. The surgical technique required for pocket preparation is as easy and provided there is adequate local anesthesia and sedation, no more painful than the prepectoral pocket [31]. The concerns regarding excessive bleeding and damage to nerves, muscle and ribs appear unfounded [31]. There is, however, genuine concern about the theoretical difficulties to be encountered at pulse generator replacement. From experience obtained as a result of pacemaker and ICD recalls, the surgical technique is a little

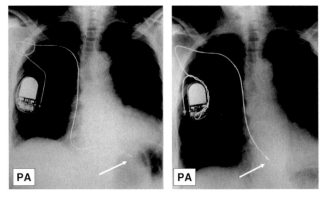

Figure 3.3 Pacemaker twiddler's syndrome. *Left:* The postero-anterior (PA) chest radiograph immediately post-implant shows the unipolar lead correctly posioned at the apex of the right ventricle (white arrow). The header block of the single chamber pulse generator lies medial. *Right:* PA chest radiograph some weeks later showing the lead retraction into the right atrium (white arrow), the tight coil of lead around the pulse generator and now the header block lies lateral.

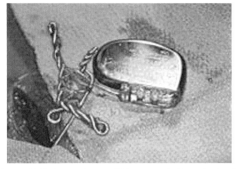

Figure 3.4 Pacemaker twiddler's syndrome. This example is a single chamber bipolar pacing system showing the tightly coiled ventricular lead at surgery.

longer and more difficult, but the final cosmetic result is much better than the prepectoral implant.

In addition, there have been reported problems with the implant location of certain piezoelectric-vibration sensors in pulse generators. In early models, the piezoelectric crystal was welded to the inner wall of the pacemaker housing. In this situation it was sensitive to applied static pressure, such as during respiration, when the can lies in the subpectoral position or directly over a rib. In contrast, in accelerometer devices which are used today, the crystal is incorporated into the hybrid circuit board and thus will not experience this problem [33].

The final decision regarding the pulse generator or ICD pocket will depend on the implanter's familiarity with implant techniques. However, in the patient with little subcutaneous tissue, serious consideration should be given to the routine use of the subpectoral pocket.

CHAPTER 4

Epicardial or epimyocardial pacing

In the adult patient with appropriate anatomy, a carefully placed transvenous, endocardial passive-fixation or active-fixation lead may be superior to a lead positioned by the epicardial approach. Although the left ventricle may be accessible using an epicardial approach, even minimally invasive techniques may be technically difficult in the post-surgical congenital heart with extensive epicardial fibrosis and adhesions. Although previously, transvenous leads had better survival rates than those implanted by the epicardial approach, today the two groups are comparable [34].

Epicardial or epimyocardial leads are generally used only when the transvenous endocardial route is contraindicated, such as following endocarditis or where there is no vascular access to the venous ventricle such as in patients with tricuspid atresia, mechanical tricuspid valve prosthesis or occluded venous channels [35].

The epicardial lead as its name implies is typically attached to the epicardium with sutures and by definition, does not penetrate the myocardium. Such a design is the platinized, porous-platinum, button-shaped, steroid-eluting electrode, which can be duplicated into a bipolar configuration (CapSure® Epi models 4965/4968, Medtronic Inc. Minneapolis, MN, USA) (Figures 4.1, 4.2). Such leads, correctly attached may give outstanding long-term pacing thresholds and sensing [36], but like all leads attached to the epicardial surface, they are prone to conductor fracture, especially in growing patients or following abdominal trauma.

In contrast, the epimyocardial lead penetrates the myocardium and may be a helical or barb design. Such leads permit adequate electrode-tissue interface contact in instances of epicardial fat or fibrosis. An alterative implant approach in patients with excessive epicardial fibrosis or fat is placement of a transvenous lead into the intramyocardial tissue via a stab incision [37].

On occasion, a permanent pacemaker or ICD is required in an adult patient with congenital heart disease, at the time of open heart surgery.

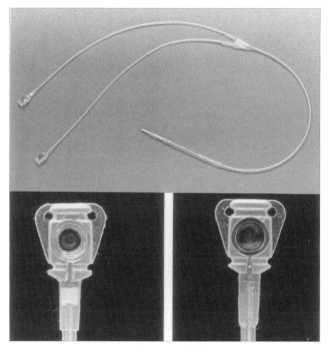

Figure 4.1 Epicardial lead. Platinized, porous-platinum, button-shaped, steroid-eluting electrodes. (CapSure® Epi model 4968, Medtronic Inc., Minneapolis, MN, USA, reproduced with permission.) *Above:* Bipolar configuration. *Below: Left* – Cathode. *Right* – Anode.

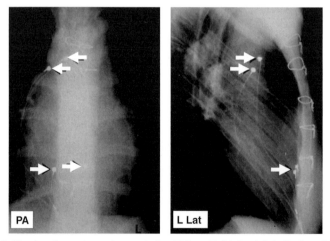

Figure 4.2 Chest radiograph, postero-anterior (PA) and left lateral (L Lat) of a adult patient with congenitally corrected L-transposition of the great vessels showing two bipolar CapSure® Epi model 4968 epicardial leads, one set on the atrium and another on the ventricle implanted after transvenous leads were extracted following bacterial endocarditis. The white arrows point to the leads.

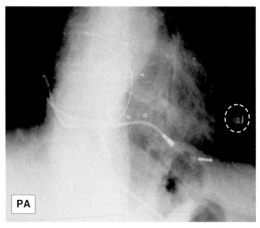

Figure 4.3 Postero-anterior (PA) chest radiograph of an adult patient with a transvenous bipolar tined lead inserted at the apex of the right ventricle at the time of tricuspid valve replacement. The lead was positioned in the ventricle first, via a purse string in the atrium and the sewing ring of the valve covers the lead as it traverses the annulus. The lead loops in the pericardium, before it passes into the anterior abdominal wall. On the extreme right, is an old fractured epicardial lead (broken circle).

Where possible, a standard transvenous lead should be placed onto the endocardial surface of the atrium and ventricle. The leads can be inserted via a purse-string ligature or a needle puncture and sheath into the right atrial appendage or body depending on the site of pulse generator, and then positioned in the right atrium [38] and ventricle [39]. Such leads can be passive-fixation or active-fixation. For better long-term results, a passive-fixation lead may be more desirable, but with positioning in the right ventricular outflow tract, an active-fixation lead will be preferable.

A similar approach is recommended for permanent ventricular pacing during insertion of a prosthetic tricuspid valve. Prior to sewing in the valve, the lead can be positioned on the endocardial surface of the ventricle, using the approach just described via the atrium. The sewing ring of the valve will then cover the lead as it traverses the annulus (Figure 4.3).

In patients, not undergoing open-heart surgery and venous access to the right-sided chambers is impossible, transvenous leads can be positioned in the right atrium and ventricle through the right atrial appendage, which is approached through a small skin incision and resecting the third or fourth costal cartilage [40,41]. The pleura is reflected and the pericardium opened. To allow fluoroscopic lead manipulation through the right atrial appendage, an introducer is held in place by a purse-string suture. The pulse generator pocket can be created through the original incision.

CHAPTER 5

Problems with right ventricular apical pacing

Pacing from the apex of the right ventricle alters the interventricular and intraventricular impulse conduction and thus distorts biventricular contractility. This may result in cellular remodeling and the development of histopathologic changes which over time adversely affects both left ventricular diastolic and systolic function [42]. This has been clearly demonstrated in the canine model [43] and more recently in long-term studies commenced in the young [44,45].

The cumulative amount of right ventricular apical stimulation as determined from stored pacemaker data has also been shown to result in corresponding levels of heart failure hospitalization and atrial fibrillation [46]. This concept of right ventricular apical pacing adversely affecting left ventricular performance has resulted in a number of recent recommendations for patients requiring pacing [47] and this is particularly important in young adults with congenital heart disease.

Although there is no doubt that the right ventricular apex should be avoided in most patients, there is still no consensus, where the preferable site is or if there is a universal "pacing sweet spot" for all patients. Congenital heart anatomy, intrinsically, can distort ventricular function and patients with congenitally corrected L-transposition of the great vessels have a morphologic "left" ventricle as the venous pulmonary pumping chamber.

The site currently considered for endocardial ventricular pacing is the right ventricular outflow tract and in particular the septal region [47]. The hypothesis is that pacing in this area creates a more physiologic depolarization pattern and theoretically better hemodynamics, less remodelling and possibly less mitral regurgitation. Based on this, right ventricular septal pacing may reduce the long-term detrimental effects of traditional right ventricular apical pacing.

Another site considered is direct His–bundle pacing. This site would obviously allow normal depolarization of the ventricles via the

His–Purkinje system. However, the site could only be used when there is no evidence of conduction tissue disease. In such patients, who are likely to have sick sinus syndrome, normal atrio-ventricular conduction would be encouraged thereby minimizing ventricular pacing and hence the site of ventricular depolarization becomes irrelevant. There is one group of patients, however that would potentially benefit from direct His–bundle pacing. This group is the one with uncontrolled atrial fibrillation and normal atrio-ventricular conduction who is being considered for His bundle ablation and should not be paced from the right ventricular apex.

Although direct His–bundle pacing has been used, nevertheless, there are a number of significant issues that prevent this from becoming a recommended ventricular implant site [48,49]. There are no commercially-available pacing lead designs that lend themselves to achieve optimal performance in this location. It is currently very difficult and time consuming to successfully directly pace the His bundle with a standard active-fixation lead. There must be a narrow QRS complex and obviously no evidence of atrio-ventricular block. In theory, the screw must penetrate the His bundle. There is debate as to whether the same conduction sequence can be achieved from pacing the surrounding para-Hisian tissues. In general, the stimulation thresholds are generally high with His bundle pacing and there is always the fear of high threshold exit block in a pacemaker-dependent patient.

Despite being recognized for a long time, there has been very little definitive work on the long-term effects of right ventricular septal pacing compared to apical pacing. This is partly due to a lack of a uniform definition of the anatomical landmarks, where it is best to position the leads and the availability of suitable leads and delivery tools [47,50,51]. Many authors refer to all leads positioned in the outflow tract as being on the septum, but clearly this is not so with many of the leads lying on the anterior or free walls. Guidelines using fluoroscopic images and ECG criteria have been published, but their accuracy has yet to be established (Figures 5.1, 5.2) [52].

The recommendation that can be made at this time for adults with congenital heart disease requiring ventricular pacing is that those patients in whom pacing was initiated in childhood, such as congenital atrioventricular block or following surgical interruption of the conduction system, will generally require many decades of pacing. That alone may contribute to contractility problems associated with the typical pacing-induced intraventricular conduction delays and intraventricular conduction changes. Such patients, will have had their initial management with a pediatric cardiologist or surgeon, and when entering adulthood, will eventually

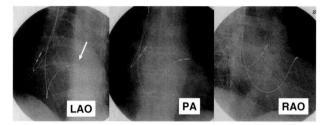

Figure 5.1 Chest cine fluoroscopic views; postero-anterior (PA), 40° left anterior oblique (LAO) and 40° right anterior oblique (RAO) of a dual chamber pacing system with the right ventricular active fixation lead in the outflow tract. In the LAO view, the ventricular lead tip (white arrow) faces posterior suggesting that the lead lies on the septum.

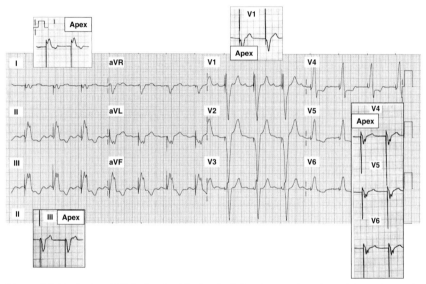

Figure 5.2 Twelve lead ECG showing bipolar dual chamber pacing with atrial sensing and pacing from the right ventricular outflow tract. The QRS is a left bundle branch block configuration, negative in I and positive in III and V4 to V6. The negative QRS in I suggests septal pacing. The axis is therefore inferior and the wave of depolarization is close to the base of the heart. In contrast, the aforementioned ECG leads are compared to unipolar ventricular pacing from the apex of the right ventricle (Apex), where the axis is superior and the wave of depolarization from the apex.

require surgery by an adult cardiologist, which may include lead replacement. Other patients may exhibit intrinsic problems with ventricular function such as L-transposition of the great vessels, irrespective of any pacing-induced cellular changes, which can further contribute to early deterioration.

It is clear, however, that whatever the group, right ventricular pacing must not be detrimental to left ventricular performance. Right ventricular apical pacing may or may not be optimal, depending on existing congenital heart anatomy and associated implanted prosthetic materials which may alter normal contractility. For instance patients, following repaired ventricular or endocardial septal defects, may have calcified patch material and fibrotic tissue extending along the septum which can effectively preclude any lead attachment in that area. In addition, the prosthetic material may hinder normal septal contractility. In such patients, the apical region may be a more effective implant site [53].

Alternative sites, such as right ventricular outflow pacing, particularly in the septum, may prove to be more effective [54]. However, it cannot always be determined where the lead actually lies in the outflow tract. The same principles apply for ICD leads, although the actual positioning is not as critical if ventricular pacing is avoided.

The detrimental effects of ventricular pacing should also be considered when programming the implanted device. In patients with sick sinus syndrome, it may be possible to use only atrial pacing. If a ventricular lead has also been implanted, the atrioventricular delay should be extended to create *minimal ventricular pacing*. A number of algorithms are available from most pacing companies to search for atrioventricular conduction and thus minimize ventricular pacing. One new algorithm uses a new dual chamber pacing mode which is essentially AAI(R). Failure to conduct to the ventricle is immediately recognized and the pacemaker automatically switches mode to dual chamber pacing (AAIsafeR™, Symphony DR 2250, ELA Medical, Cedex, France and EnRhythm™ P1501DR Medtronic Inc., Minneapolis, MN, USA). This mode of pacing is useful in patients with prolonged or varying PR intervals, where it may be difficult to stretch the atrioventricular delay to encourage ventricular sensing.

CHAPTER 6

What type of lead fixation device do I use?

Transvenous leads may be passive-fixation or active-fixation. The predominant passive-fixation design uses soft flexible tines positioned immediately behind the electrode (Figure 6.1). Correctly positioned in either the atrium or ventricle, these leads have very low dislodgement rates and because there is little endocardial irritation, the chronic stimulation thresholds are very low, particularly with steroid-elution [55–57]. Although these leads are ideal for chronic endocardial pacing, the absence of an active-fixation device usually limits their application to traditional pacing sites.

It must also be remembered that in the typical post-surgical congenital heart patient, the right atrial appendage may be missing or rudimentary from previous bypass cannulation. In addition, in congenitally corrected L-transposition of the great vessels, the right-sided ventricle has a

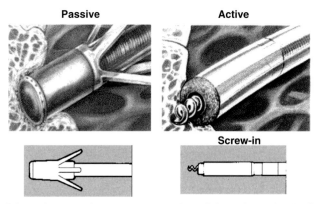

Figure 6.1 Schematic comparing transvenous endocardial passive and active fixation leads. *Left:* Passive fixation lead with four tines, which when implanted in the right ventricle lie beneath and between trabeculae. *Right:* Active fixation lead with extendable and retractable helical screw.

"left" ventricular morphology, which may preclude effective tined lead positioning beneath or between trabeculae.

Early model active-fixation leads, particularly in the atrium, had high, unacceptable stimulation thresholds [58]. However; the newer steroid-eluting screw-in designs have acceptable acute and chronic performance in both the atrium [56] and ventricle [59, 60]. Of particular importance to the young pacemaker recipient is that modern active-fixation leads can now have a thin diameter and be virtually isodiametric, making lead extraction, if necessary, easier (see Figure 7.5, p 27). Steroid-eluting active-fixation leads have also been shown to perform well in the right ventricular outflow tract with marginally better long-term stimulation thresholds compared to the apex [61].

Unless the pacing leads are to be positioned in traditional sites in structurally normal hearts, active-fixation pacing leads are preferable in patients with adult congenital heart disease requiring permanent cardiac pacing [62].

CHAPTER 7

Consider steerable stylets or catheters

An adult patient with congenital heart disease may present unique challenges to the implanter and in particular, negotiating obstacles to position leads in almost inaccessible sites. To aid lead-positioning in such situations, two types of delivery systems have been developed.

The steerable stylet (Locator® Model 4036, St Jude Medical, Minneapolis, MN, USA) (Figure 7.1) has been available for a number of years and found to be useful in a variety of troublesome clinical situations, unique to congenital heart diseases. One particularly helpful situation is positioning the atrial lead onto the roof of the left atrium in patients who have undergone the Mustard intra-atrial baffle procedure for D-transposition of the great vessels. The distal curve is ideal in placing the lead tip at the medial portion of the roof well away from the phrenic nerve and thus preventing nerve stimulation which is the most common post operative complication in this group of patients. This will be discussed further in Chapter 20.

Ironically this narrow distal curve is the major disadvantage of the steerable stylet as it is not particularly helpful in turning corners in enlarged chambers or reaching the right ventricular outflow tract. Figure 7.2 shows three different stylet curves in identical pacing leads. The Locator® has a very narrow curve excellent for atrial appendage and the aforementioned left atrium. The J stylet is the typical atrial appendage shape and the curved stylet is useful in negotiating large chambers. In Figure 7.3, the Locator® lies in the body of a huge left atrium and was of little value in negotiating the lead into the right ventricle, via a tricuspid valve annuloplasty ring for "belt and braces" pacing (Chapter 8).

The steerable stylet concept of the Locator® has been shown, on occasions to be very useful in negotiating the lead along venous channels, particularly on the right side. This is because the stylet can be inserted straight and once in the chamber, the steerable curve can be applied. In contrast, stylets with fixed curves may not enter the brachiocephalic or

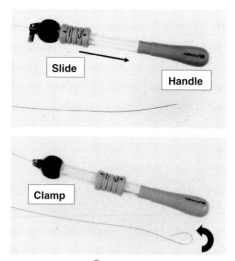

Figure 7.1 The steerable stylet (Locator® Model 4036, St Jude Medical, Minneapolis, MN, USA). Reprinted with permission from St Jude Medical. *Above:* The stylet is straight. *Below:* The slide is pulled down towards the proximal part of the handle and the stylet curves into a tight U shape. When the stylet is fully inserted into a lead, the clamp at the distal end of the handle attaches to the lead connector and can be removed from the handle to allow the stylet to be partially removed.

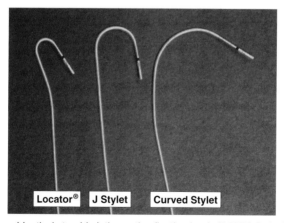

Figure 7.2 Three identical steroid eluting active fixation leads (1488T, St Jude Medical), with three different stylets inserted. From the left, the lead with Locator® has a small sharply angled curve suitable for positioning the lead in certain circumstances, but unsuitable in large chambers. The advantage to the Locator® is that the curve can be created from the straight position without removing the stylet. In the center, the preformed atrial J stylet allows the lead to enter the atrial appendage or attach to the atrial wall. The curved stylet on the right has been fashioned to allow the lead to negotiate enlarged chambers. Reprinted with permission from St Jude Medical.

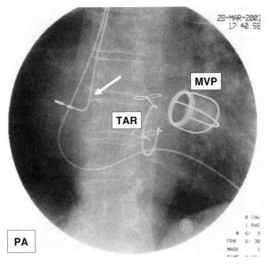

Figure 7.3 Postero-anterior (PA) chest cine fluoroscopic view to show two ventricular leads (belt and braces) being inserted in a patient with a tricuspid annuloplasty ring (TAR) and torrential tricuspid regurgitation. There is marked right atrial and ventricular chamber enlargement. One lead passes through the annuloplasty ring to the apex of the right ventricle. The other lead (white arrow) lies in the body of the right atrium. The operation of the Locator® produces only a small change in the distal curvature and does not help in lead advancement through the annuloplasty ring. The broad stylet curve shown in Figure 7.2 was required. There is a ball and cage mitral valve prosthesis (MVP).

innominate vein toward the heart, but rather proceed retrograde towards the arm in the axillary vein or up into the neck in the internal jugular vein (Figure 7.4). Although this can usually be prevented by not peeling the introducer until the curved or J stylet has been inserted, it does on occasion prevent the appropriate stylet from being used and can be overcome with a Locator®.

The Locator® stylet is only manufactured for the active-fixation leads of that company and may not reach the tip of either the active or passive-fixation leads of competitors. As a consequence, the lead tip may not respond to the desired curve, thus limiting its efficacy.

An alternative to the steerable stylet is a steerable catheter (SelectSite®, Medtronic Inc.) through which a thin 4.1F lumenless fixed screw active-fixation lead (SelectSecure® Medtronic Inc.) can be passed (Figures 7.5, 7.6). Such a pacing system has application in adults with congenital heart disease such as Ebstein's anomaly or in patients, following the Mustard and Fontan [63] procedures. In these situations, the leads are expected to follow obscure pathways and to traverse stenosed baffles and shunts [64].

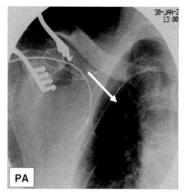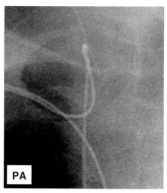

Figure 7.4 Postero-anterior (PA) chest cine fluoroscopic views to demonstrate the usefulness of the Locator®, particularly on the right side. *Left:* The atrial lead with the J stylet passes into the axillary vein toward the arm. Although a straight stylet followed by a J stylet would probable be effective, nevertheless a steerable stylet would allow the passage of the lead and positioning in the right atrial appendage (white arrow) without stylet exchange. *Right:* During the stylet exchange for right atrial appendage positioning, the atrial J stylet pushes the lead up into the internal jugular vein. This can be a troublesome complication of atrial lead implantation.

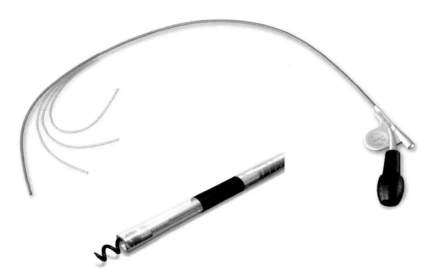

Figure 7.5 Steerable catheter (SelectSite®, Medtronic Inc.). At the distal end, four views of the catheter are shown demonstrating the range through which the catheter can be steered. In the center is the thin 4.1F lumenless fixed screw active-fixation lead (SelectSecure® Model 3830 Medtronic Inc.) which can be passed through the steerable catheter. Reproduced with permission from Medtronic Inc., Minneapolis, MN, USA.

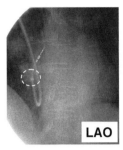 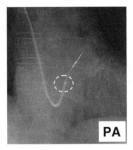 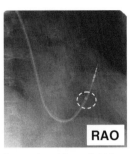

Figure 7.6 Chest cine fluoroscopic views from the left; 40° left anterior oblique (LAO), postero-anterior (PA) and 40° right anterior oblique (RAO). A steerable catheter (SelectSite®, Medtronic Inc.) is in the right ventricular outflow tract and an active fixation lead is being positioned on the septal wall. The distal end of the catheter is highlighted with the broken circle.

Other potential uses for the steerable stylet are negotiating enlarged chambers and positioning leads in alternate pacing sites in the right atrium and ventricle. An added advantage is the thinner lead diameter which potentially may also prevent recurrent obstruction seen with standard larger diameter leads, particularly across intravascular stents.

CHAPTER 8

Safety in numbers – the belt and braces technique

There is always concern when pacemaker implantation or revision is performed in a pacemaker-dependent or potentially dependent patient. A solution is the *belt and braces* technique, where two leads are positioned in the right ventricle and connected to the pulse generator [65]. This is particularly helpful in patients with torrential tricuspid regurgitation, where during surgery the active-fixation lead is seen to dislodge and prolapse with great force into the right atrium. If the patient is pacemaker dependent, a second ventricular lead should be implanted to act as a backup (Figures 7.3, 8.1). Most of these patients will be in chronic atrial fibrillation and the two leads can be connected to a dual chamber pulse generator programmed DDD(R).

The aim of pacemaker programming is to provide ventricular pacing from the atrial channel followed by sensing in the ventricular channel. In order to achieve this, the programming should provide a non-rate adaptive AV delay of about 120 ms and safety pacing turned off (Figure 8.2). Because of the possibility of atrial channel T wave sensing, mode switching,

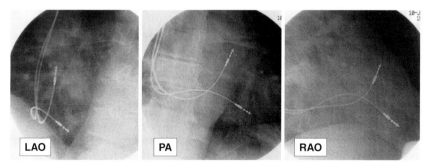

Figure 8.1 Chest cine fluoroscopic views from the left; 40° left anterior oblique (LAO), postero-anterior (PA) and 40° right anterior oblique (RAO) demonstrating belt and braces dual site pacing. Two leads are implanted in the right ventricle; one at the apex and the other in the right ventricular outflow tract.

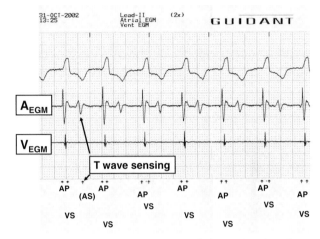

Figure 8.2 Guidant (Guidant Inc. Minneapolis MN, USA) dual chamber electrograms demonstrating intermittent T wave sensing in a patient with dual site pacing. From above, ECG lead II, atrial electrogram (A_{EGM}), ventricular electrogram (V_{EGM}) and event channel. The pacemaker has been programmed DDDR with a non-rate adaptive AV delay of 120 ms, which results in right ventricular outflow tract pacing from the atrial channel (AP) followed by right ventricular apical sensing in the ventricular channel (VS). In the atrial electrogram, the T wave is intermittently sensed in the post ventricular atrial refractory period [(AS)].

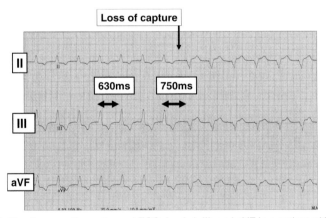

Figure 8.3 Simultaneous three channel ECG, leads I, III, and aVF in a patient with dual site ventricular pacing undergoing atrial (right ventricular outflow tract) stimulation threshold testing at 95 bpm (630 ms). There is ventricular pacing from the right ventricular outflow tract lead and sensing from the right ventricular apical lead. When loss of capture occurs, there is a 120 ms delay and pacing from the right ventricular apical lead commences. Note the change in QRS axis demonstrating the ECG configuration with pacing from the two ventricular sites. See Figure 5.2.

which is not relevant, should also be inactivated. Should the lead connected to the atrial channel dislodge, then the other lead will automatically and immediately provide pacing. The system can be tested using the *atrial threshold test*. At atrial threshold, the lead attached to the ventricular port paces after the set AV delay (Figure 8.3).

In the rare situation, where the patient is still in sinus rhythm, a biventricular pacemaker can be used. A model must be chosen that can accept a bipolar IS-1 lead into the left ventricular port or a special adapter used. Once connected, dual site right ventricular pacing (equivalent to biventricular pacing) can be utilized. If necessary, at a later stage, when the lead thresholds are stable, one of the ventricular channels can be programmed OFF.

CHAPTER 9

Do old leads need extraction?

One of the difficulties occasionally encountered in adults with congenital heart disease is the problem of having to insert new transvenous leads in a patient who already has old implanted hardware. A decision must be made as to the risks and benefits of lead extraction prior to implantation. The longer the original leads have been implanted, the more fibrotic are the endocardial tunnels in which they are embedded and consequently the more difficult and hazardous the extraction. Although leads implanted less than four years have a 95% successful extraction rate, that success rate drops to about 80% for leads implanted for over 10 years [66]. The final decision will also depend on the skill and experience of the extractor, the number of leads implanted and the remaining venous channels.

CHAPTER 10

Stenosed venous channels

In patients with previously implanted pacing and ICD leads, who require new leads, venous stenosis is a common problem. The stenosis will invariably lie close to the original venous entry site, making subclavian or even axillary puncture difficult and on occasion, impossible. The stenosis may continue all the way to the right atrium and is not always a reflection of the number of leads present in the venous system. Even single leads may result in significant stenosis. If the ipsilateral side is to be used for the new lead, it is desirable to always obtain a venogram preoperatively (Figure 10.1).

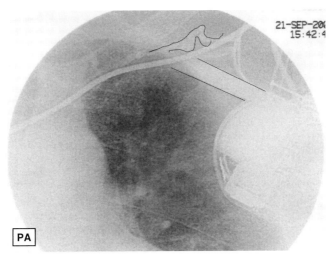

Figure 10.1 Postero-anterior (PA) left-sided venogram to show venous occlusion around the pacing leads. The proximal axillary-subclavian vein is outlined as is one of the large collaterals around the thrombosis site. In this case, the subclavian was entered and a Glidewire® passed along the vein to the superior vena cava. Using a number of dilators, the vein became large enough to accept an introducer.

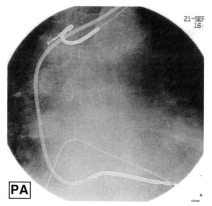

Figure 10.2 Chest cine fluoroscopic postero-anterior (PA) view demonstrating a new ICD lead caught at the brachiocephalic (innominate)-superior vena caval junction in a patient who had a nonfunctioning ICD lead that required replacement.

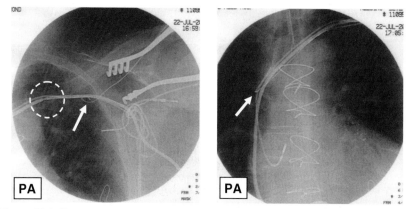

Figure 10.3 Chest cine fluoroscopic postero-anterior (PA) views demonstrating the passage of a Glidewire® to the heart. *Left:* The white arrow points to the coiled end progressing along the vein parallel to the fractured ICD lead (broken circle). *Right:* The Glidewire® has now passed into the superior vena cava (white arrow). In this example, a standard introducer guide wire could not be passed.

If the contralateral side is to be used, then it can be assumed that a passageway to the superior vena cava will be present. If obstruction is encountered, then a venogram is best performed at surgery allowing better definition of the site of the stenosis. If the contralateral side is successfully used, the question remains as to whether the original implanted pulse generator should be removed or not. Any operative procedure carries the risk of infection and if the pulse generator is comfortable then it should be left intact and used as temporary back-up pacing until the power source depletes. Follow-up testing should also be carried out on the original pulse generator because of the potential problem of loss of sensing.

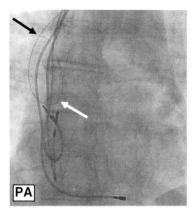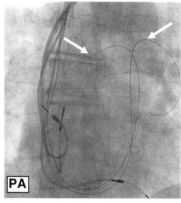

Figure 10.4 Chest cine fluoroscopic postero-anterior (PA) views demonstrating the passage of a Glidewire® into the pulmonary artery from the left side. The pacemaker dependent subject has three pacing leads from the right side. Only one of the atrial leads is functioning. The ventricular lead has a high stimulation threshold and impedance. Rather than try lead extraction, an attempt was made to pass two new pacing leads from the left side. *Left:* The wire has passed to the upper-right atrium (white arrow), where it has coiled back with the tip in the superior vena cava (black arrow). Great difficulty was experienced passing it into the body of the right atrium. *Right:* Two Glidewires® have now been passed into the right ventricle and lie in the left and right pulmonary arteries (white arrows). Attempts at lead placement are shown in Figures 10.7–10.9.

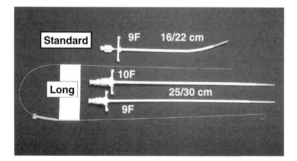

Figure 10.5 Venous introducer sets (Di-Lock, St Jude Medical). Reprinted with permission from St Jude Medical. *Above:* Standard 9 French (9F) introducer with 16 cm cannula and a 22 cm dilator. *Below:* Long 9 and 10 French (9F, 10F) introducers with 25 cm cannula and a 30 cm dilator.

Even when significant stenosis is encountered on the ipsilateral side, pacing and ICD leads can still be inserted. A standard subclavian puncture should be attempted aiming the needle under fluoroscopic control to the area where venous flow was seen on the venogram. Particularly on right-sided implants, if a standard subclavian puncture fails, then the tip of the needle should be positioned more medial, just beyond where the

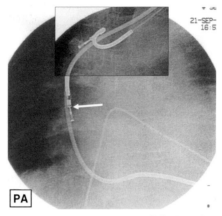

Figure 10.6 Chest cine fluoroscopic postero-anterior (PA) view of the same case as Figure 10.2. Using a long introducer, the lead has been passed beyond the brachiocephalic (innominate)-superior vena caval junction and now passes easily into the right atrium.

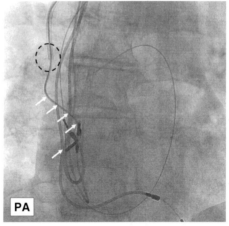

Figure 10.7 Chest cine fluoroscopic postero-anterior (PA) view of the same case as Figure 10.4. The tip of the long introducer (black broken circle) has been passed almost to the junction of the superior vena cava and right atrium. Through this introducer the lead has been passed into the mid right atrium (five white arrows) but cannot progress further. The procedure was abandoned on the left side.

previously implanted leads turn to enter the brachiocephalic or innominate vein. The vein at this point is often large and patent because of the confluence of the jugular and subclavian veins.

Even after successful venous puncture and entry, it is often very difficult to get a standard stiff introducer guide wire or pacemaker lead into the right atrium. The vein is thickened with narrowings or shelves on which the

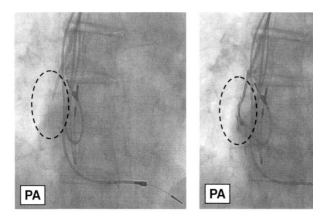

Figure 10.8 Chest cine fluoroscopic postero-anterior (PA) views of the same case as Figures 10.4 and 10.7. *Left:* The long introducer has now been passed from the right side and the tip lies in the upper right atrium (black broken circle). Right: A venogram shows a very narrow passageway through the right atrium due to probable extensive thrombosis and fibrosis (black broken circle).

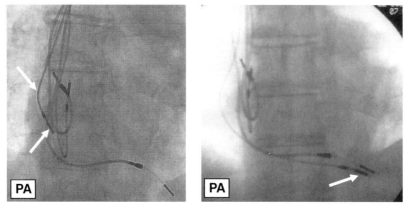

Figure 10.9 Chest cine fluoroscopic postero-anterior (PA) views of the same case as Figures 10.4, 10.7 and 10.8. *Left:* A ventricular active-fixation lead has been passed through the long introducer and lies near the floor of the right atrium (white arrows). *Right:* The ventricular lead has been passed with much difficulty to the apex of the right ventricle below the original lead (white arrow).

guide wires or leads get caught (Figure 10.2). A stiff guide wire may perforate the vein and enter the mediastinum and even the pericardium, resulting in acute retrosternal pain. To prevent such a scenario, it is desirable to use a very floppy 80 cm Glidewire® discussed in Chapter 2 (Figure 2.1). Unlike stiff guide wires, the Glidewire® can often easily negotiate troublesome angles and flip over fibrous shelves (Figures 10.3, 10.4).

Once the guide wire is in the atrium or beyond, an introducer can be inserted. Frequently, both the intra and extra vascular areas are fibrotic and difficult to negotiate. When encountered, the implanting physician can pass the dilator or trocar along the channel to create a pathway. A range of smaller or larger size dilators can be used to finally create a smooth pathway for the introducer. The final introducer may need to be 1F larger than the recommended size for the proposed lead. Standard introducers are usually about 16 cm long and may not traverse the brachiocephalic-superior vena cava junction. When the lead is passed through and lies beyond the cannula, it may get caught on a shelf or within a stenosis at this junction (Figure 10.2). Longer introducers (25 cm) are available and multiple sizes should be kept in reserve for such situations (Figure 10.5).

Using the Glidewire® and a range of long dilators and introducers, it is surprising how successful it is to pass the new lead to the heart in what was originally thought to be an impossible situation (Figure 10.6).

Figures 10.4 and 10.7–10.9 highlight the value of the Glidewire® and long introducers. This case study is of a pacemaker-dependent patient in whom three leads have been previously passed to the heart using venous entry sites on the right side. A new ventricular lead was required and a decision made to implant a new dual chamber system on the left. In Figure 10.4 (left), the Glidewire® cannot pass beyond the upper part of the right atrium. After much manipulation, the wire and then a second Glidewire® are passed to the pulmonary artery followed by a long introducer which lies almost at the junction of the superior vena cava and right atrium (Figure 10.7). An active-fixation lead can be passed only to the mid-right atrium. The left side was abandoned and using a right subclavian puncture and Glidewire®, a long introducer is passed this time to the right atrium as the passageway is shorter. A venogram reveals thrombosis within the right atrium (Figure 10.8). An attempt is made once again to pass the active-fixation lead and this time after much manipulation, the lead can be passed to the right ventricular apex and secured (Figure 10.9). Without the Glidewire® and long introducer, the procedure would have failed, necessitating a potentially dangerous lead extraction or epimyocardial leads.

CHAPTER 11

Use of the coronary venous system

Pacing of the ventricle via the coronary venous system has long been practiced, although in the majority of the earlier cases, lead placement in the middle or lateral cardiac veins was inadvertent and unrecognized at the time of implantation [67]. More recently there have been reports of ventricular pacing from the cardiac venous system, in patients, where there was failure to place the lead in the right ventricle, such as in the presence of a persistent left superior vena cava or a mechanical tricuspid valve prosthesis [68–73].

With the recent development of specifically designed coronary sinus delivery systems, thin pacing leads can now be successfully positioned on the epicardial surface of the left ventricle. Although such techniques are usually reserved for biventricular pacing, nevertheless, the technique has specific applications in adult congenital heart disease, particularly in situations where there is no or limited access to the venous ventricle.

Before coronary sinus cannulation is considered in adults with congenital heart disease, it should be remembered that the venous drainage of the heart into the right atrium may not be normal. In particular, a left superior vena cava will result in marked difficulties in trying to achieve left ventricular pacing. The incidence of this abnormality draining into the coronary sinus is about 3–5% of patients with structurally abnormal hearts [74]. In turn depending on the presence or absence of a bridging brachiocephalic or innominate vein, and certain repaired congenital heart defects, the coronary sinus may be absent or significantly enlarged. In very rare situations, the coronary sinus may not communicate with the right atrium, but rather drain into the left subclavian vein via a left superior vena cava [75]. By cannulation of these vessels a left ventricular lead was successfully implanted for biventricular pacing. An enlarged thebesian valve within the coronary sinus may obstruct the ostium making lead positioning difficult or impossible.

In patients with D-transposition of the great vessels who have undergone Senning or Mustard procedures which involves the insertion of an intra-atrial baffle, the coronary sinus is obviously not accessible from the venous system.

There is also a rare atrial septal defect located at the typical position of the coronary sinus ostium. In this anomaly, the coronary sinus itself may be absent. An additional defect can be found in the coronary sinus-left atrial wall (unroofed coronary sinus), causing both left and right atrial shunting. These defects occur early in embryogenesis due to abnormal sinus venosus development. Since the existing shunt may be small, the defect may not be detected until later in life.

On rare occasions the coronary sinus may be absent or atretic. In these instances, commonly associated with right atrial isomerism (right atrial duplication with absent left atrial development), enlarged thebesian veins particularly from the left side provide myocardial venous drainage to the right atrium. Longitudinal partitioning of the coronary sinus into two lumens with different venous drainage has also been successfully used for placement of a left ventricular lead [76].

The coronary sinus may be inaccessible from the right atrium following corrective cardiac surgery. This may occur following the closure of a large atrial septal defect. In such a situation, the coronary sinus may open into the left atrium. Similarly, following corrective surgery of Ebstein's anomaly, the coronary sinus may lie on the ventricular side of the tricuspid valve prosthesis.

When anatomical confusion remains as to the presence or origin of the coronary sinus, careful review of any operative or previous cardiac catheterization notes is essential. Computerized tomographic imaging, magnetic resonance imaging or two dimensional echocardiography with color doppler may also help (Figure 11.1). As a last resort, a coronary angiogram and follow through may assist in defining the course of the coronary sinus [75]. Table 11.1 summarizes the possible abnormalities in the coronary sinus position in congenital cardiac abnormalities, both pre and post operatively.

The technology involved in pacing the left ventricle via the coronary sinus is rapidly evolving, but implantation is still subject to a number of recognized complications such as high threshold exit block, phrenic nerve stimulation, and late lead dislodgement. At this time, the technique would only be recommended in a non-pacemaker-dependent patient, although adults with congenital atrioventricular block and poor left ventricular function should be strongly considered for biventricular pacing.

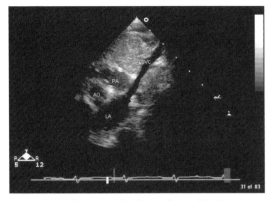

Figure 11.1 Suprasternal two-dimensional echocardiographic view demonstrating a left superior vena cava (LSVC), commmunicating directly with the left atrium (LA) in a pateint with an atrial septal defect. The coronary sinus is absent. The aorta (AO) and pulmonary (PA) arteries at the level of the valves are indicated.

Table 11.1 Possible abnormalities of the coronary sinus in congenital heart disease.

Pre-operative congenital heart disease	Possible abnormality
Atrial septal defect Common atrium Right atrial isomerism	Absent coronary sinus Left superior vena cava drains to left atrium
Unroofed coronary sinus	Atrial septal defect Coronary sinus drains to both right and left atria
Persistent left superior vena cava	Absent or dilated coronary sinus Coronary sinus drains into left subclavian vein
Univentricular heart	Stenosis of the coronary sinus ostium Unroofed coronary sinus
Wolff-Parkinson-White	Coronary sinus diverticulum
Interrupted inferior vena cava	Hemiazygous vein drainage to left superior vena cava
Ebstein's anomaly	Unroofed coronary sinus Coronary sinus ostium on ventricular side of valve
Fontan repair (Univentricular heart)	Dilated tortuous coronary sinus
Intra-atrial baffle repair (D-transposition of the great vessels)	No venous access to coronary sinus

CHAPTER 12

Consider growth in teenagers

Although this text deals with congenital heart disease in the adult patient, nevertheless, the implanting physician may, on occasion, be referred a growing teenager for pacemaker or ICD implantation. In this situation, screw-in leads should be positioned and looped to add extra length to the intravascular lead [77]. As the teenager grows, the extra loop of lead is gradually resorbed (Figure 12.1). Too large a loop, however, may not be desirable. In the right ventricle it may cause cardiac arrhythmias, whereas, in the atrium, the loop may position itself across the tricuspid valve and become entangled and subsequently attached to the valve mechanism. As the teenager grows, severe tricuspid regurgitation may result.

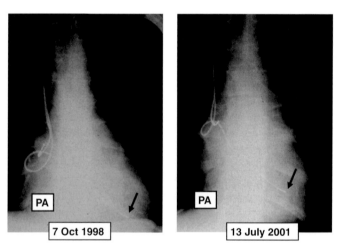

Figure 12.1 Postero-anterior chest radiographs taken 33 months apart in a growing teenager. At implantation, a large loop was left in the ventricular lead as it traversed the right atrium. Unfortunately, this loop also incorporated the atrial lead, which resulted in that lead pulling the ventricular lead upwards and out of the ventricular apex. The arrows point to the ventricular lead tip.

Leaving the redundant loop outside the vein in the pacemaker pocket has also been suggested. The lead is secured to the tissues via the lead collar, using slowly absorbable suture material. The lead can then be drawn into the intravascular path as the teenager grows, especially in the 13–17 age group where more vertical growth can be anticipated.

PART 2

Patients, principles and problems

For convenience, adult patients with congenital heart diseases can be divided into:
- Those who have not required heart surgery so far in their lives
- Those who have undergone previous corrective or palliative cardiac surgery
- Those in whom there is no venous access to the ventricle (Table P 2.1).

Table P2.1 Classification of adult congenital heart disease.

No previous cardiac surgery
  Pacemaker/ICD required
    Congenital atrioventricular block
    Congenitally corrected L-transposition of the great vessels
    Congenital long QT syndromes
  Pacemaker/ICD a challenge
    Atrial septal defects and patent foramen ovale
    Persistent left superior vena cava
    Dextrocardia
    Ebstein's anomaly
Previous corrective or palliative cardiac surgery
    D-transposition of the great vessels
    Septal defects including tetralogy of Fallot
    Ebstein's anomaly
No venous access to ventricle
    Univentricular heart

SECTION A

No previous cardiac surgery: pacemaker/ICD required

CHAPTER 13

Congenital atrioventricular block

First described by Morquio over 100-years ago [78], congenital atrioventricular block is defined as being present at birth [79]. However, not all cases are diagnosed at this time and therefore, atrioventricular block detected later, without evidence of myocarditis, trauma or any other etiological factors or the presence of other coexisting congenital malformations of the heart, should be regarded as congenital atrioventricular block, particularly if there is a familial incidence.

There are also a number of other reported conditions associated with congenital bradycardia syndromes. These include idiopathic and progressive fibrous degeneration of the conduction system in the young, long QTc syndromes and sodium channelopathies. Recent studies of mutations in the sodium channel gene SCN5A, have shown a heterogeneity of congenital bradycardia syndromes associated with normal cardiac anatomy and atrioventricular block [80]. An association of the SCN5A gene mutation has also been reported with progressive atrioventricular conduction tissue fibrosis, as in the Lev-Lenegre syndrome [81]. In addition to the well-established long QTc-associated mutations, familial bradycardia syndromes of atrial bradycardia or standstill and prolonged H–V conduction time may present at any age requiring atrial or ventricular pacing [82,83]. As knowledge of these genetically inherited conditions predisposing to bradyarrhythmias and heart block unfold, it is imperative that the implanting physician be aware of their existence and thus plan therapy and in particular the need for an ICD rather than a pacemaker.

Pathologically, in congenital atrioventricular block, the interruption in conduction occurs between the atrium and the conducting system distal to it, usually at the bundle of His or within an aberrant conducting system [79,84]. When the interruption occurs at the atrial level, the deficiency lies in the atrial musculature, although the atrioventricular node may be deficient, absent or abnormal [85,86]. If the interruption is more distal, then it usually occurs in the penetrating portion of the bundle of His with the more distal bundle and its branches either normal or defective [79,87,88]. An aberrant conducting system may result in absent bundle branches [87,89] or an anterior accessory conducting system and this is usually associated with a ventricular septal defect. In this situation the block usually occurs as a result of ongoing fibrosis and hemorrhage [79].

His bundle electrograms confirm the pathological findings. In most cases the block is proximal to the bundle of His, although in some cases split His potentials have been recorded [90–92]. Such conduction abnormalities may occur in normal hearts or are associated with other congenital abnormalities, particularly atrioventricular or ventricular septal defects or congenitally corrected L-transposition of the great vessels. Similar conduction abnormalities may also be present in cases of apparent congenital complete atrioventricular block that appears in adulthood [93].

As in the original description by Morquio [78], there may be a strong familial incidence, which can be divided into two groups; congenital or adult onset [94]. In the adult onset form, the electrocardiograph may show varying degrees of bundle branch block in family members [78,89,95–97]. By monitoring the ECG, it may therefore be possible to predict which family members will require permanent cardiac pacing at a later age [94]. An increased incidence of conduction disorders in the relatives of patients with high degree atrioventricular block has also been reported [89,98]. A relationship between congestive cardiomyopathy and cardiac conduction abnormalities presenting in the fourth and fifth decades and investigated in a family over six generations confirmed a hereditary basis to the heart block, which was clearly not congenital [99].

A number of other congenital syndromes may present with cardiac conduction disorders during the late teens or adulthood. This includes the Holt-Oram syndrome which involves upper limb abnormalities and congenital heart lesions such as atrial and ventricular septal defects. Conduction disturbances include sinus arrest [100] and heart block [101]. The Kearns-Sayre syndrome is a triad of progressive external ophthalmoplegia, retinitis pigmentosa and atrioventricular block [102–104], although sick sinus syndrome has also been reported [105].

The incidence of congenital complete atrioventricular block is approximately 1:22,000 live births [106]. The pathogenesis may be either abnormal embriogenic molding as described earlier or maternal collagen disease. In the latter, maternal immunoglobulin G antibodies to the soluble ribonucleoproteins SS-A/Ro and SS-B/La, cross the placental barrier during the first trimester and interact with the fetal cardiac antigens involved in the development of the atrioventricular node, fibrous body, and annulus

[107,108]. The subsequent inflammatory reaction results in necrosis of the developing conduction tissue and replacement with fibrous tissue.

These antibodies have been reported with systemic lupus erythematosus, rheumatoid arthritis, scleroderma, and Sjogren's syndrome [109, 110]. Up to 98% of mothers whose offspring have congenital atrioventricular block can be shown to have these antibodies [111], although many of the mothers demonstrate no symptoms or signs of the auto immune disease at the time of gestation [112]. Not all offspring in mothers with systemic lupus erythematosus develop congenital atrioventricular block, although high antibody titers and a previous pregnancy complicated by congenital atrioventricular block are sensitive predictors of risk [113].

As stated earlier, not all cases of complete heart block in the young are due to a congenital interruption of the proximal conducting system. Other causes such as myocarditis, trauma or even congenital tumors such as a mesothelioma of the atrioventricular node have been described [114]. A subset of patients with congenital atrioventricular block is prone to development of a cardiomyopathy as part of their genetically inherited condition [115]. An association of a congenital aneurysm of the membranous septum has also been reported [116].

The challenge for the physician, referred a young adult with complete atrioventricular block is, when to implant a permanent pacemaker. Provided the patient has no symptoms, the ventricular rate, particularly with exertion is satisfactory, no ventricular tachyarrhythmias are documented and the echocardiograph and chest radiograph remains within normal limits, the patient can be followed regularly without implantation of a permanent pacemaker. Any deterioration in these parameters fulfills the indication for permanent pacing (Figure 13.1).

For adults, the 24-hour Holter ambulatory monitor plays an important role. Heart rates less than 40 beats per minute with pauses up to three seconds when awake and five seconds when asleep are likely to result in symptoms (Figures 13.2, 13.3). Not surprisingly, asymptomatic patients have significantly higher ventricular rates than symptomatic patients and ventricular rates decrease with age [117]. Previous reports have indicated which patients are at risk to develop bradycardia related symptoms [118]. Ventricular bradycardia with resting atrial rates greater than 150 bpm suggests neurohumoral responses to developing adverse physiology. Permanent ventricular pacing is recommended to prevent deterioration in left ventricular function. Frequent complex ventricular ectopy, particularly overnight, even in the absence of ventricular tachyarrhythmias, may be an early indicator of sudden death or emerging left ventricular dysfunction [119,120].

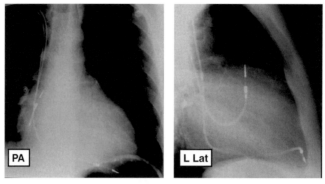

Figure 13.1 Congenital atrioventricular block. Chest radiograph of a symptomatic 26-year old male with congenital complete heart block corrected with dual chamber pacing. Note the considerable cardiomegaly.

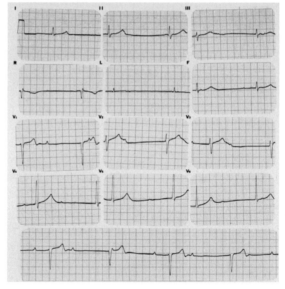

Figure 13.2 Congenital atrioventricular block. Resting 12-lead ECG showing congenital complete heart block with a narrow QRS. Note there is also mild sinus bradycardia, necessitating rate adaptive dual chamber pacing.

With the development of reliable long-life dual chamber pacing systems which are usually easy to implant with few complications, there has been a tendency to implant the permanent pacemaker "sooner than later". This is very different from the early pacing experience, when the pacemaker longevity was relatively short and the complication rate high. Most adolescents with congenital complete heart block on entering adulthood

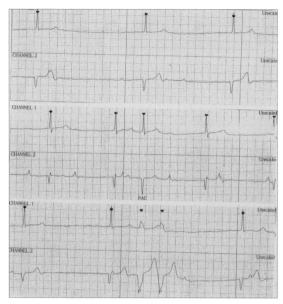

Figure 13.3 Congenital atrioventricular block. Twenty-four hour, two channel Holter monitor recording from the same patient with congenital complete heart block seen in Figure 13.2. *Top line:* Ventricular rate is 25 PPM. Note the slow sinus rate. *Middle line:* A premature atrial complex (PAC) probably represents atrioventricular conduction with marked first degree atrioventricular block. *Bottom line:* Ventricular couplet.

will eventually develop symptoms and consequently receive a permanent pacemaker [117,121]. Not surprisingly, permanent pacing has been recommended to all patients older than 15 years [122].

In certain clinical situations, it remains prudent to recommend implantation of a permanent pacemaker even in the "asymptomatic" patient. For instance, there may be sporting or occupational reasons for this recommendation. Another situation of particular importance is the young female planning a family. The stress of pregnancy may result in symptomatic acute hemodynamic deterioration during the second and third trimester and following delivery. This may occur in about 40% of patients [122]. There is nothing worse for both patient and implanting physician, than the emotional stress of an urgent permanent pacemaker implantation in a pregnant patient shrouded in lead from the diaphragm down. Following physiologic pacing, in an otherwise normal female, there is no contraindication to pregnancy [123] and no special precautions are required at delivery, unless in the unlikely circumstances, a minute ventilation sensor has been programmed ON. If cautery is to be used, such as with a planned or urgent cesarean section, then the sensor should be programmed OFF. Bacterial endocarditis prophylaxis is probably not indicated, but is generally given.

Despite the recent tendency to implant permanent pacemakers, there are case reports in the literature of successful follow-up without pacing for up to 40 years even with documented Stokes-Adams episodes [124, 125]. However, other reports document sudden death in young adults with abnormalities of the conduction system [126]. There are also rare reports of improvement in conduction with age [124,127].

Provided there are no other congenital cardiac abnormalities present, the implantation of a permanent cardiac pacemaker should be a routine procedure. A number of principles apply:

• The routine use of epicardial leads requiring a thoracotomy is not indicated.

• In the adult, provided the patient is in sinus rhythm, reestablishment of atrioventricular synchrony is essential.

• In some centers, a single pass lead VDD system is preferred. In this situation, it is critical to establish that sinus node function is normal. Sinus bradycardia or a suboptimal sinus response to exertion may occur with complete atrioventricular block in the young adult [94]. With modern atrial leads being so reliable, it is just as easy to implant a two lead system as it is to implant a single pass VDD lead. Another advantage of the two lead system is the ability to place the ventricular lead in the high right ventricular outflow tract, preferably on the septum.

• To avoid excessive intravascular hardware, extremely thin leads implanted using steerable catheters should be considered, particularly, in the young.

• For cosmetic reasons, the pulse generator should lie as deep as possible. In patients with little adipose tissue a subpectoral pocket should be considered.

A question now being asked is whether left ventricular or biventricular pacing should be considered in the young patient with congenital atrioventricular block. In a highly symptomatic patient with an ejection fraction <30%, this would fulfill standard indications for this therapy. In two recently published multi-center reports of children and young adults with congenital heart disease receiving biventricular pacing for myocardial dysfunction, including patients with congenital heart block, biventricular pacing did prove to be effective in improving symptoms and function [128, 129]. However, in patients with normal or reasonable left ventricular function, there is no evidence that this would either improve symptoms or prognosis. Indeed the complexity of the procedure, the added complications and the reduced pulse generator longevity, should prevent the implanting physician from using cardiac resynchronization therapy at this stage of its development.

At the other end of the spectrum, young patients with congenital heart block and normal ventricular function have been shown to require only ventricular pacing [130]. In this situation, optimization of the ventricular lead placement in the right ventricular outflow tract to provide the best contractility is desirable [52]. This situation is unlikely to be encountered in the adult patient.

CHAPTER 14

Congenitally corrected L-transposition of the great vessels

Complete atrioventricular block will eventually occur in about 15–20% of patients with congenitally corrected or levo (L)-transposition of the great vessels [131], and is statistically the most important congenital malformation associated with atrioventricular block [132]. In this congenital abnormality, there are both atrio-ventricular discordance and ventriculo-arterial discordance. Simply explained, the normal heart has concordance: a morphologic "right" atrium drains into a right-sided morphologic "right" ventricle, which then gives rise to the pulmonary artery.

In congenitally corrected L-transposition of the great vessels, the embryologic heart tube bends or loops to the left instead of the right, yet the great arteries develop normally. This inverts all the structures derived from the bulboventricular part of the heart, which includes the atrioventricular valves, the ventricles and the proximal part of the great arteries; hence the terms levo or L-transposition and ventricular inversion. The result is that a normally positioned right atrium connects to a right-sided ventricle with "left" ventricular morphology, which in turn ejects blood into a normal pulmonary artery. Pulmonary venous blood enters a normally positioned left atrium, drains into a left-sided ventricle with "right" ventricular morphology and ejects blood to the circulation via the aorta (Figure 14.1). The blood flow pattern is thus normal and there is no cyanosis as compared with D-transposition of the great vessels. Consequently, there is discordance between the atria and ventricles and between the ventricles and great arteries. This leftward ventricular looping also distorts the great vessels, so that the aorta lies anterior to the pulmonary artery. On the right side, an anatomic "left" ventricle drains into a posterior rather than an anterior pulmonary trunk (Figures 14.2).

In the normal heart, the atrioventricular node develops as a posterior structure, whereas with congenitally corrected L-transposition, there are both anterior and posterior atrioventricular node structures with the His bundle arising anterior [131]. The absence, arrested development

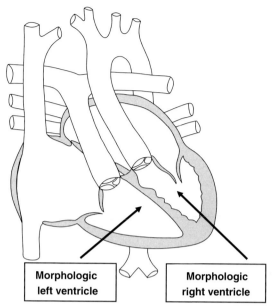

Morphologic
left ventricle

Morphologic
right ventricle

Figure 14.1 Congenitally corrected L-transposition of the great vessels. With congenitally corrected L-transposition of the great vessels, the anatomic difference is a levo (L) – looping of the embryonic cardiac tube such that the ventricles are reversed. The venous right sided ventricle has "left" ventricular smooth wall morphology and the arterial left ventricle "right" ventricular trabecular morphology. The aorta attaches to the morphologic right ventricle and lies anterior. The pulmonary artery attaches to the posterior pulmonary trunk with blood flowing posterior.

or destruction of this anterior conducting system can give rise to complete atrioventricular block at any time during life [133–135], with cases reported as old as 65 years [136]. Therefore, it would not be surprising that an undiagnosed adult case of congenitally corrected L-transposition of the great vessels presents with high degree atrioventricular block and the unsuspecting implanter could then be confronted with a previously unseen radiological and implant dilemma. Indeed, it is worth remembering that any young or even middle aged person with complete heart block should have an echocardiograph prior to pacemaker implantation to exclude congenitally corrected L-transposition of the great vessels.

The implantation of a pacemaker in a patient with congenitally corrected L-transposition of the great vessels is not difficult, provided the anatomy is understood. For the experienced implanter, it may even be easier than the normal implant. The reasons for this are related to the position of the interventricular septum. As shown in Figure 14.2, the ventricles lie to the

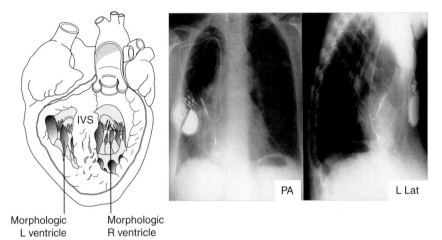

Morphologic   Morphologic
L ventricle   R ventricle

Figure 14.2 Congenitally corrected L-transposition of the great vessels. *Left:* Schematic to show the relationship of the ventricles and the interventricular septum (IVS) which lies in an antero-posterior plane. This is unlike the normal heart where the septum traverses from left to right with the right ventricle lying anterior. This positioning of the septum is very important when viewing the position of the ventricular lead. *Middle:* Postero-anterior (PA) chest radiograph to show the positioning of a ventricular pacemaker lead at the apex of the morphologic left ventricle. Note how the ventricular lead fits into the schematic and therefore does not need to turn right to reach the ventricular apex. *Right:* Left lateral (L Lat) chest radiograph to show the ventricular lead passing anterior.

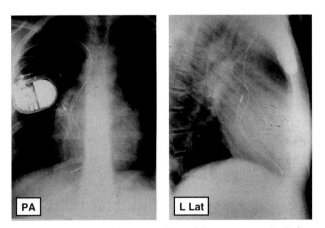

Figure 14.3 Congenitally corrected L-transposition of the great vessels. *Left:* Postero-anterior (PA) chest radiograph to show the positioning of a ventricular pacemaker lead at the apex of the morphologic left ventricle. Note how the ventricular lead at the apex turns right rather than left and this fits the schematic shown in Figure 14.2. *Right:* Left lateral (L Lat) chest radiograph to show the ventricular lead passing anterior.

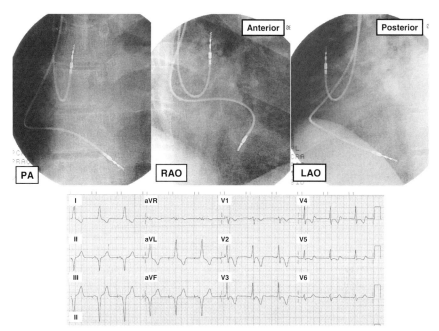

Figure 14.4 Congenitally corrected L-transposition of the great vessels. *Above left:* Chest cine fluoroscopic postero-anterior (PA) view to show the positioning of a ventricular pacemaker lead at the apex of the morphologic left ventricle. In this case right sided ventricular chamber is dilated and the lead passes to the left as in a normal right ventricular implant. *Above middle and right:* Right (RAO) and left (LAO) anterior oblique views to show the lead lying posterior. *Below:* Resting 12-lead ECG from the same patient demonstrating dual chamber pacing with an inferior axis and the characteristic tall R waves from V2 to V6.

side of each other whereas in the normal, the right lies anterior to the left ventricle. The septum is thus antero-posterior rather than left to right.

With pacemaker implantation, the atrial lead is positioned normally, but depending on the size of the ventricular chambers, their orientation and the way they sit on the diaphragm, the fluoroscopic course of the ventricular lead may not turn sharply medial and to the left to traverse the atrioventricular valve. Rather the lead passes inferior through the valve to the apex of the right sided but anatomic left ventricle. The subsequent fluoroscopic views may confuse the implanting physician, leading to prolonged implantation times, even though there is virtually no resistance to lead placement. In addition, since this venous ventricle has smaller trabeculae, active-fixation leads may be preferable.

Figure 14.2 shows the ventricular lead passing inferior without a bend as if into the floor of the right atrium and fits nicely with the accompanying schematic. Depending on its position in the ventricle, the lead tip may

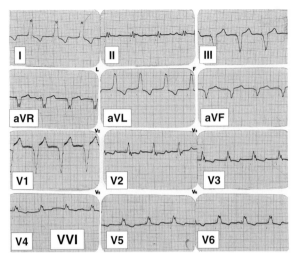

Figure 14.5 Congenitally corrected L-transposition of the great vessels. Resting 12-lead ECG of the dual chamber pacing system shown in Figure 14.3 programmed VVI to demonstrate ventricular pacing. The axis is inferior and there are dominant R waves from V2 to V6 suggesting left ventricular pacing.

lie anterior or posterior on the left lateral radiograph (Figure 14.2). It is this appearance that raises the concern about lead dislodgement, because of the relative lack of an extensive trabecular network in the morphologic left ventricle [137]. However, even with old style leads, there was no increased incidence of lead dislodgement and this would be consistent with the necropsy findings of sufficient trabeculation to entrap tined leads [138].

Another appearance is shown in Figure 14.3. Here the ventricular lead passes to the right, which also fit nicely into the schematic (Figure 14.2). In this case, the left lateral confirms the anterior position of the lead. This appearance would mimic dextrocardia, to be discussed later, but the passage of the leads on the right and the position of the atrial lead confirm ventricular inversion. A third example is shown in Figure 14.4. In the postero-anterior view, the lead appears to pass normally to the left side, although the right and left anterior oblique views confirm a posterior position of the lead tip in the ventricle. This example probably has an enlarged right sided ventricle and the differential diagnosis is placement of the lead in the middle cardiac vein via the coronary sinus.

The pacemaker electrocardiographic appearances of congenitally corrected L-transposition are quite characteristic. The paced QRS complexes show a bundle branch block appearance with a dominance of left ventricular forces as if the left ventricle lies on the right side. The ECG may

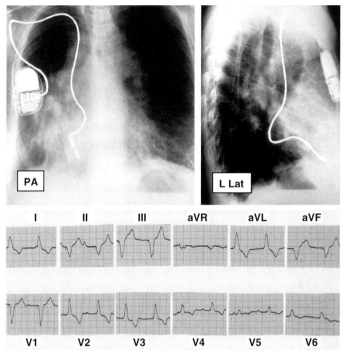

Figure 14.6 Patient with a normal heart lying to the right following a right lobectomy for tuberculosis many years ago. *Above left:* Postero-anterior (PA) chest radiograph showing the ventricular lead passing straight down into the right ventricle in a similar fashion to the patient with congenitally corrected L-transposition of the great vessels shown in Figures 14.2 and 14.3. This is because the ventricles have moved to the right to fill the space left by the pneumonectomy. The lead has been highlighted. *Above right:* Left lateral (L Lat) chest radiograph to show the ventricular lead passing anterior. *Below:* Twelve Lead ECG of the single chamber ventricular pacing system shown above. There is VVI pacing with the axis inferior and tall R waves are present from V2 to V6. This is an identical situation to that shown with congenitally corrected L-transposition of the great vessels, but on this occasion it is a normal right ventricle that is paced.

be similar, wherever the lead lies in the right sided ventricle (Figures 14.4 and 14.5). Of interest, the ECG and chest radiographic appearances are almost identical to a situation where the lead lies at the apex of the right ventricle, but the heart has moved markedly to the right; because of a previous right lower lobectomy for tuberculosis (Figure 14.6). It is quite obvious that congenitally corrected L-transposition of the great vessels presents little challenge to the implanting physician provided the anatomy is understood.

CHAPTER 15

Congenital long QT syndromes

In the era prior to ICDs, it became fashionable to implant a single chamber atrial or dual chamber pacemaker programmed with an atrial low rate of 80–90 ppm in patients with congenital long QT syndromes, with or without atrioventricular block [139–142]. This, together with intensive beta blockade was often successful in preventing ventricular ectopic activity and hence, torsade de pointes. In general, beta blockade alone or together with left cervical thoracic sympathectomy, failed to control serious life threatening symptoms. In some cases, beta blockade was contraindicated because of side effects or the beta blocker induced bradycardia acted as a provocative agent for torsade de pointes [142]. Although both atrial and ventricular pacing have been shown to shorten the mean QT interval, it doesn't however, alter the mean corrected QT interval [142].

A number of mechanisms have been postulated to explain the success of pacing for the congenital long QT interval. This includes:
• Decreasing the dispersion of refractoriness preventing critically timed premature ventricular ectopic activity from causing reentry ventricular tachyarrhythmias [143],
• Reducing automaticity [144],
• Preventing bradycardia-induced afterpotentials [145].

What type of pacemaker should be implanted? In theory, the objective should be to increase the heart rate by atrial pacing alone, thus avoiding implanting a ventricular lead that could encourage ventricular irritability, although, today this would be unusual, because of the thinner, less rigid pacing leads used [140]. However, as discussed earlier, there have been sporadic reports of atrioventricular block with hereditary long QT interval [140, 142, 146, 147]. Thus a dual chamber system, programmed to avoid ventricular pacing should be considered (Figure 15.1). The prevalence of atrioventricular block in congenital long QT interval is unknown, although its occurrence suggests prolonged refractoriness in the conducting system [142]. Once initiated in childhood, patients

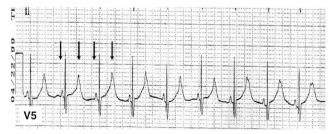

Figure 15.1 ECG rhythm strip, lead II demonstrating second degree AV block in a patient with long QTc syndrome. The black arrows point to the p waves.

with congenital long QT syndromes can be expected to require life-long pacing.

Although pacemakers can still be used to prevent symptoms in patients with congenital long QT syndromes, nevertheless in the adult patient, the hardware today, must also incorporate an ICD. Provided there are no congenital cardiac malformations present, the implantation procedure is standard.

No previous cardiac surgery: pacemaker/ICD a challenge

CHAPTER 16

Atrial septal defects and patent foramen ovale

A patent foramen ovale is the most frequently found congenital abnormality of the heart and results from the normal fetal circulation persisting post natal. An incidence of 27% in otherwise normal hearts has been reported with the incidence falling with advancing age, but still as high as 20% in the elderly [148].

Atrial septal defects are also one of the most common congenital defects occurring in adults with a familial incidence well known to cardiologists. Within this group are patients who have added electrical abnormalities including prolonged atrio-ventricular conduction, high degree atrio-ventricular block, sudden death and the need for permanent pacing [149–154].

In general, an isolated atrial septal defect (Figure 16.1) or patent foramen ovale, whether in the young or later in life, presents no impediment to a standard pacemaker or ICD implantation. However, to the unsuspecting implanting physician, the atrial and or ventricular leads may cross the atrial septum through a defect [155, 156] or a patent foramen ovale [156–162] and be implanted in the left atrium or ventricle resulting in an increased risk of systemic embolization, such as stroke [156] or amaurosis fugax [157, 159]. Asymptomatic cases, diagnosed many years later have been reported [155, 161]. In general, once systemic embolization occurs, removal of the leads are recommended either transvenously [158] or in open heart surgery [157, 159, 162]. Even in asymptomatic cases, anticoagulation with warfarin (coumadin) is recommended if the leads are not removed [156]. Transthoracic [157–159, 161, 162] and transesophageal echocardiography [155, 156] as well as computerized tomography [160] are very helpful in diagnosis of lead malpositioning across the atrial septum.

An example of left ventricular pacing as a result of the lead crossing a patent foramen ovale is demonstrated in Figure 16.2. The high arching of the lead with its summit sitting across the atrial septum is characteristic and should alert the implanting physician, who should then review the

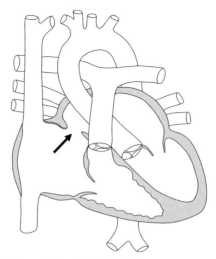

Figure 16.1 Schematic of an atrial septal defect in the more common central or "secundum" position (black arrow), typically in the area of a patent foramen ovale. Other less common locations include a high opening near the superior vena cava (sinus venosus defect) and an opening along the septal region of the tricuspid valve (primum defect).

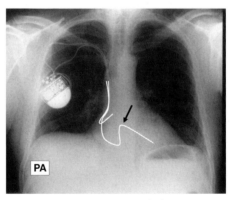

Figure 16.2 Patent foramen ovale. Postero-anterior (PA) chest radiograph of a ventricular pacing lead traversing a patent foramen ovale and attached to the apex of the left ventricle. The black arrow points to where the lead crosses the atrial septum. The appearance is characteristic of a lead in the left ventricle. The intra cardiac portions of the atrial and ventricular leads are highlighted.

ECG to determine which ventricle is being paced (Figure 16.3). A clue is the inability to pass the lead to the right ventricular outflow tract. Because of the risk of systemic emboli, the lead should be withdrawn to the right atrium and correctly positioned. This should also be performed if detected at a later date. The lead position can be confirmed by echocardiography (Figure 16.4).

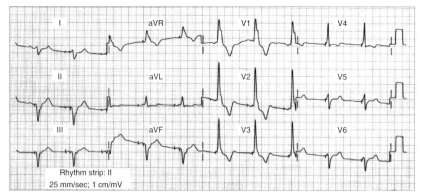

Figure 16.3 Patent foramen ovale. Twelve lead ECG from the same patient as in Figure 14.1 showing dual chamber pacing with a right bundle branch block appearance indicating left ventricular pacing.

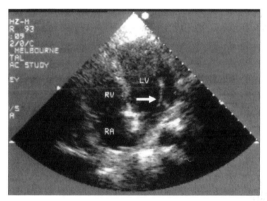

Figure 16.4 Patent foramen ovale. Apical four chamber two dimensional echocardiograph demonstrating a pacing lead passing from the left atrium via the mitral valve towards the left ventricular (LV) apex (white arrow). On the left is the right atrium (RA) and ventricle (RV). This is the same case shown in Figures 16.2 and 16.3.

Once a pacing lead has crossed a septal defect or foramen ovale, the question remains as to whether the inter-atrial connection should be closed to prevent paradoxical embolism. The decision would depend on the size of the shunt, age of the patient, previous emboli and the experience of the institution in closing such shunts. The advent of transvenous delivery of closure devices has greatly facilitated repair.

In the post-atrial defect closure patient, atrial lead implantation may add challenges, especially if the septum contains prosthetic patch material or a mechanical device (Figure 16.5). Septal or Bachman's bundle pacing may not be feasible due to extensive fibrosis in those areas. Also, as in

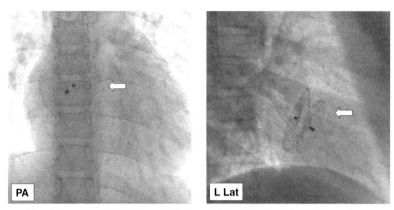

Figure 16.5 Postero-anterior (PA) and left lateral (L Lat) chest radiographs to demonstrate a secundum atrial septal defect closed with an Amplatzer® Septal Occluder device (AGA Medical Corporation, Minneapolis, MN, USA) shown by the arrow. Device diameters vary according to defect opening. This device measures 24 mm. Potential difficulty of lead placement at a septal location is obvious.

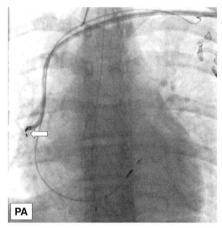

Figure 16.6 Postero-anterior (PA) chest radiograph demonstrating atrial lead placement along the atrial superior vena cava junction (arrow) to approximate the sinus node region utilizing the steerable catheter delivery system (SelectSite®, Medtronic Inc.), which permits acute angulation even in small atria.

any post bypass patient, the appendage stub may not accommodate atrial passive fixation leads. A recent report of successful atrial pacing from the sinus node region adds promise as that area of the right atrium is typically free of fibrosis [163]. The introduction of the steerable catheter delivery system as indicated previously greatly facilitates lead implant in that region (Figure 16.6).

CHAPTER 17

Persistent left superior vena cava

Embryologically, the left superior vena cava represents a persistence of the left anterior and common cardinal veins (Figure 17.1). Normally after birth, these structures are atretic and are represented as the ligament and small vein of Marshall on the left atrium, which in turn drains into the coronary sinus. The incidence of persistent left superior vena cava is about 0.5% [164], but is more frequent when associated with other congenital heart abnormalities [165]. When a left superior vena cava persists, it descends into the chest parallel to the right superior vena cava and drains into the right atrium via a markedly dilated coronary sinus. In most cases, a right superior vena cava is also present, but in about 0.05% it may be absent leaving a single huge left vena cava [166]. (Figure 17.2). Despite the large congenital abnormality, most cases of isolated persistent left superior vena cava are asymptomatic, hemodynamically insignificant and may be found inadvertently at autopsy, cardiothoracic surgery or when attempting to pass a pacemaker or ICD lead to the heart. An association with sick sinus syndrome and other conduction tissue disorders has been reported [167,168].

The abnormality is encountered more frequently in pacemaker implanters who use the left side. When the right side is used and a right superior vena cava is present, the implanting physician may be unaware of the abnormality. As discussed in Chapter 11, on very rare occasions, the coronary sinus may be unroofed leading to a right to left shunt resembling an atrial septal defect. Another very rare congenital malformation is direct drainage of the left superior vena cava into the left atrium. In both instances, the pathology would not be relevant to the adult cardiologist.

Encountering a left superior vena cava during a pacemaker implantation can be a very challenging experience with well-described specific operative techniques to position the ventricular lead. Not surprisingly the early literature reported unsuccessful attempts at transvenous lead placement, thus necessitating the epi/myocardial approach [169–171]. The challenge

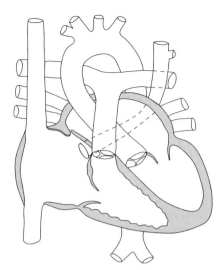

Figure 17.1 Schematic of a persistent left superior vena cava draining into the coronary sinus. Failure of left superior cardinal vein regression, typically associated with absence of innominate vein development, allows for venous drainage into the right atrium.

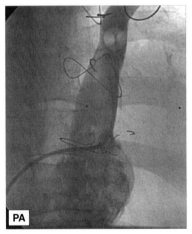

Figure 17.2 Persistent left superior vena cava. Chest cine fluoroscopic postero-anterior (PA) view of a venogram demonstrating a very dilated coronary sinus associated with persistence of a left superior vena cava and absent innominate vein. Difficulty of pacing lead insertion through such a chamber into the right ventricle can be anticipated.

for the pacemaker implanter is to negotiate the wide tortuous passage-way through the left superior vena cava and coronary sinus into the right atrium and then the lead must make a sharp turn to cross the tricuspid valve, if necessary bouncing off the lateral atrial wall (Figures 17.3–17.5). This is achieved by creating a loop using a variety of different shaped

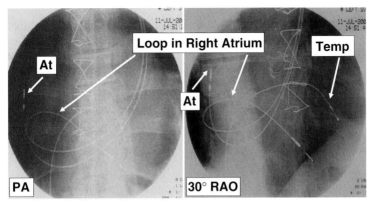

Figure 17.3 Persistent left superior vena cava. Chest cine fluoroscopic postero-anterior (PA) and 30° right anterior oblique (RAO) views to show the ventricular lead emerging from the coronary sinus looping in the right atrium and then passing to the floor of the right ventricle. The atrial lead (At) lies against the lateral wall of the right atrium. There is a temporary lead (Temp) from the femoral vein in the right ventricle.

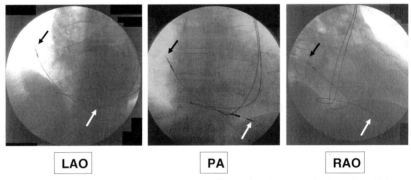

Figure 17.4 Persistent left superior vena cava. Chest cine fluoroscopic views from left to right, left anterior oblique (LAO), postero-anterior (PA) and right anterior oblique (RAO) to show the ventricular lead emerging from the coronary sinus, looping in the large right atrium and passing through the tricuspid valve to the floor of the right ventricle (white arrow). The atrial lead is attached to the lateral wall of the right atrium (black arrow).

curved stylets [172–175]. Once the tricuspid valve has been crossed, the lead must then be advanced into the body of the chamber using a curved stylet until contact is made with the endocardium. Lead dislodgement into the right atrium during implantation is unfortunately a frequent occurance. Figure 17.5 shows how difficult this procedure can be.

The anatomical features of the persistent left vena cava are drawn over the chest radiograph. In this case, the right atrium and ventricle were

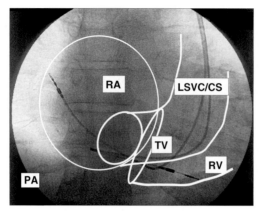

Figure 17.5 Persistent left superior vena cava. Chest cine fluoroscopic postero-anterior (PA) view of the same case shown in Figure 17.4, but with the anatomical structures of the heart drawn in. The persistent left superior vena cava and coronary sinus (LSVC/CS) is a huge venous channel that drains into a very large right atrium (RA). The tined ventricular lead is seen to emerge from the orifice of the LSVC/CS, makes a sharp turn, crosses the tricuspid valve and is implanted in the inflow tract of the right ventricle. The atrial active-fixation lead also emerges from the orifice of the LSVC/CS and passes superior to the lateral wall of the RA.

enlarged and there was moderately severe tricuspid regurgitation. By sheer chance, the tined lead became attached to the right ventricular inflow tract with excellent testing parameters.

With a persistent left superior vena cava, the ventricular pacing site is usually not chosen and wherever the lead goes is acceptable, provided the position is stable and the pacing parameters satisfactory. It is anticipated that the steerable catheter may fascilitate lead placement, although maybe not in the ventricle (Figure 17.6).

As discussed earlier, the use of active-fixation leads has been recommended for many years, because of the concerns of lead dislodgement [176]. A single pass lead [177], ICD [178, 179] and left ventricular leads for biventricular pacing [180, 181] have also been successfully inserted via a persistent left superior vena cava. In a case report of a patient with persistent left superior vena cava, the loop of lead was reversed as it emerged from the coronary sinus, so that the tip went superior into the body of the ventricle rather than to the floor and apex [182]. The active-fixation lead was then successfully attached to the bundle of His. Thrombosis of the massive coronary sinus has been reported following pacemaker lead implantation in a patient with an absent right and a persistent left superior vena cava [183].

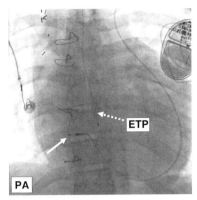

Figure 17.6 Persistent left superior vena cava. Chest cine fluoroscopic postero-anterior (PA) view of a patient with tricuspid atresia and a left superior vena cava who had previously undergone a Fontan procedure (Chapter 23). Atrial pacing was achieved via the left superior vena cava and coronary sinus using a SelectSite® steerable catheter through which a thin 4.1F lumenless fixed screw active-fixation lead (SelectSecure®) was passed to the low right atrium (white arrow). There is more flexibility in positioning this thin lead compared to a standard screw-in lead. There is an esophageal temperature probe (ETP) present (broken arrow).

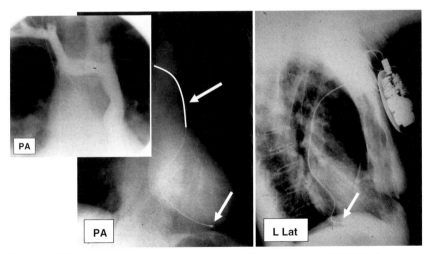

Figure 17.7 Persistent left superior vena cava. *Left:* Postero-anterior (PA) view of a venogram showing the left superior vena cava and an absent right sided vena cava. *Middle:* Postero-anterior (PA) chest radiograph. A unipolar lead from the right side (highlighted – upper white arrow) is passed into the left superior vena cava. Note that the lead does not loop in the right atrium before passing to the apex (lower white arrow). *Right:* Left lateral (L Lat) chest radiograph showing the lead passing posterior indicating that it has passed into the middle cardiac vein.

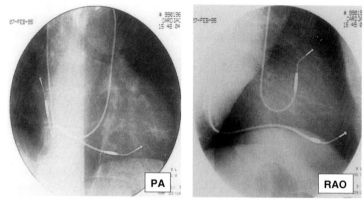

Figure 17.8 Persistent left superior vena cava. *Left:* Chest cine fluoroscopic postero-anterior (PA) view showing both left and right superior venae cavae connecting by an innominate vein. The passive-fixation ventricular lead from a right venous entry site, passes down the left superior vena cava, is looped in the right atrium and crosses the tricuspid valve and is implanted close to the apex of the right ventricle. The passive-fixation atrial lead from the same venous entry site passes down a right superior vena cava and is attached close to the right atrial appendage. *Right:* Chest cine fluoroscopic right anterior oblique (RAO) view showing the ventricular lead passing anterior to the right ventricular apex.

In a patient with a persistent left superior vena cava, the ventricular lead may not leave the coronary sinus, but rather enter a cardiac venous tributory and in this way, pace the left ventricle. This will usually be the middle or lateral cardiac vein and in the postero-anterior view will mimic the apex of the right ventricle (Figure 17.7). However, there will be no right atrial loop and the lead will lie posterior in the left lateral view. Such a position in a cardiac vein would be acceptable if the lead position and stimulation thresholds are stable. If the patient is or will become pacemaker dependent, then the implanting physician should consider a second ventricular lead with an attempt this time to place it in the right ventricle. If successful, a "belt and braces" biventricular pacing system is achieved. In the case discussed in Figures 17.4 and 17.5, there was concern about lead dislodgement and thus an attempt was made to pass an active-fixation lead into the right ventricle for a more secure attachment. Because of the right atrial enlargement, the lead could not be bounced of the atrial wall and looped into the ventricle.

If, with a left sided surgical approach, there is failure to position a ventricular lead via a persistent left superior vena cava, then it is incumbent upon the implanting physician to check for the presence or absence of a right superior vena cava (Figure 17.8). This can be attempted initially by probing from the left side or attempting a venogram. If a brachiocephalic or innominate communication between the two venae cavae does not exist, then a standard right venogram or digital subtraction angiogram is indicated [184]. Another alternative is to consider left ventricular epicardial pacing via a cardiac venous branch of the coronary sinus [185]. A case in which both venae cavae drained into a large coronary sinus and did not allow a pacing lead to enter the right atrium required epicardial pacing [186]. Congenital absence of both the left and right venae cavae has been reported [187].

In general, there is less a problem positioning a right atrial lead via a left superior vena cava. The lead enters the right atrium and with an appropriate generous curve on the stylet moves easily to the lateral wall [188] (Figures 17.3–17.6). The lead must be active-fixation and the longer "standard ventricular length" (58 cm) chosen. Unlike the normal atrial lead that hangs in the atrium, the lead may push against the atrial wall and in time may lead to signs of clinical perforation and pericardial effusion. An elective follow-up post-operative echocardiograph is mandatory.

CHAPTER 18

Dextrocardia

Dextrocardia is a positional congenital abnormality in which the cardiac apex is located on the right side of the chest (Figure 18.1). As an isolated abnormality, such as situs inversus, which is the mirror image of the normal or situs solitus where the atria are in the normal positions, pacemaker

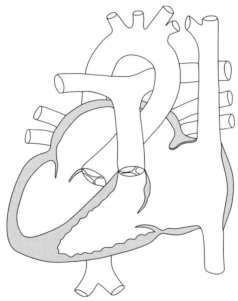

Figure 18.1 Schematic of a heart with the mirror image of situs solitus, "dextrocardia" anatomy. The atria, the ventricle and the great vessels are in a normal concordance (normally connected chambers and great vessels), but the apex is to the right instead of the left. Systemic venous return is to the left. A chest radiograph typically will show an associated right-sided stomach and left-sided liver.

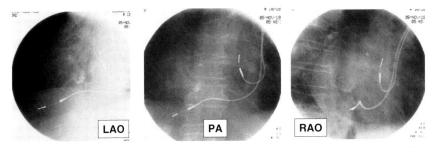

Figure 18.2 Dextrocardia. Three chest cine fluoroscopic views; left anterior oblique (LAO), Postero-anterior (PA) and right anterior oblique (RAO) demonstrating the appearance of a dual chamber pacing system in a patient with dextrocardia. The PA view is a mirror image of the normally positioned heart, whereas the LAO and RAO images are reversed.

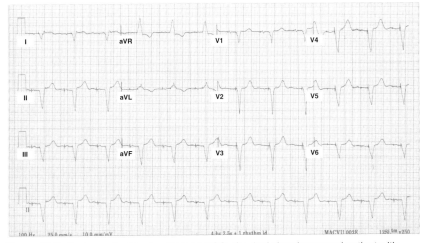

Figure 18.3 Dextrocardia. Resting 12-lead ECG of a dual chamber paced patient with dextrocardia. Compared to the normally positioned heart, lead I is upside down, leads II and III are reversed as are aVR and aVL. Because the right ventricular lead is at the apex of the right ventricle, all six chest leads show QS waves and cannot be differentiated from the normally positioned heart (see Figure 5.2). This appearance can be mimiced in the normal by reversal of the arm leads.

implantation presents no challenge to the implanting physician, once orientation has been determined (Figure 18.2). The paced ECG should also be helpful in diagnosing dexrocardia during the procedure (Figure 18.3). It should also be remembered that dextrocardia may be associated with a variety of other complicated congenital heart abnormalities involving the atria, ventricles and great vessels [62].

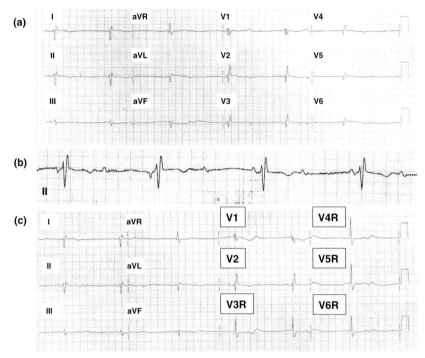

Figure 18.4 Dextrocardia. (a) Resting 12-lead ECG of a patient with dextrocardia, 2:1 atrioventricular block and partial right bundle branch block. Lead I is upside down, leads II and III are reversed as are aVR and aVL. There is no development of R waves across the anterior chest leads. (b) Rhythm strip lead II magnified to confirm the 2:1 atrioventricular block. (c) Same ECG as in A. Leads V3 to V6 are now placed across the right chest wall (R) demonstrating the normal R wave progression.

Thankfully, the pacemaker implanter is usually aware of the situation preoperatively, particularly if there are other complex lesions. If not the preoperative resting ECG would give a clue as to the orientation, provided the rhythm was not complete heart block with a wide QRS (Figure 18.4).

CHAPTER 19

Ebstein's anomaly

Ebstein's anomaly, which represents <1% of all congenital heart diseases, is of clinical importance to pacemaker physicians because many of the patients, who reach adulthood, develop bradyarrhythmias (Figure 19.1) [189]. The disorder is characterized by downward displacement of the tricuspid valve orifice so that the cusps, with the exception of the medial

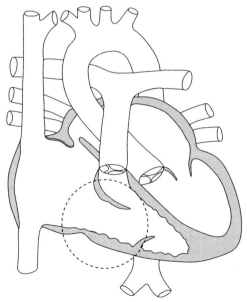

Figure 19.1 Schematic of the apical displacement of the tricuspid valve seen in Ebstein's anomaly. This results in a superior "atrialized" portion of the right ventricle, which is associated with atrial pressure, yet ventricular intracardiac electrogram recordings (broken circle).

two-thirds of the anterior cusp, originate from the right ventricular wall rather than from the tricuspid annulus [190, 191]. This displacement may be as low as the junction of the inflow and the outflow portions of the right ventricle. The displaced tricuspid valve divides the right ventricle into two parts:

• The atrialized portion which lies between the origin of the normal tricuspid annulus and the displaced tricuspid orifice.

• The remainder of the true right ventricle, which lies beyond the tricuspid valve.

The size of the atrialized portion of right ventricle varies greatly and its walls may be fibrous and paper thin or muscular and well formed. The tricuspid valve tissue is almost always redundant, wrinkled and the chordae tendineae poorly developed or absent. The actual valve orifice is generally smaller than normal and is usually incompetent [190,191].

Cardiac arrhythmias and conduction disturbances occur in 20–25% of patients with Ebstein's anomaly [192, 193], and commonly involve pre-excitation syndromes. Pacemaker therapy is necessary in about 3–4% [194]. The indications for pacemaker therapy include persistent atrial stand-still [195], atrio-ventricular block which can be de novo [196, 197], post surgery [198] or following radiofrequency ablation [199]. Due to the mor-phologic abnormalities in Ebstein's anomaly, endocardial ventricular lead placement can be challenging and in those patients who have not had surgery, there are three pacing options [200].

Pre-valve

The atrialized portion of the right ventricle, which behaves hemodynamic-ally like the right atrium, has electrophysiologic characteristics of the right ventricle. This can be used to advantage to position a transvenous ventricu-lar lead pre-valve in order to pace the right ventricle [201]. By avoiding crossing the tricuspid valve, lead-induced exacerbation of tricuspid regur-gitation can be prevented. In its severe form, the muscle in this pre-valve cul de sac may be poorly formed or absent resulting in a thin aneurysmal wall and ventricular pacing may therefore require a high voltage or the area may be electrically silent. If successful, the chest radiograph will show the ventricular lead tip to be in a postero-medial location (Figure 19.2) and the ECG reveals right ventricular pacing with a left bundle branch block configuration and a leftward or superior axis, confirming that the cathode lies against right ventricular endocardium at the most inferior aspect of the cardiac silhouette (Figure 19.3).

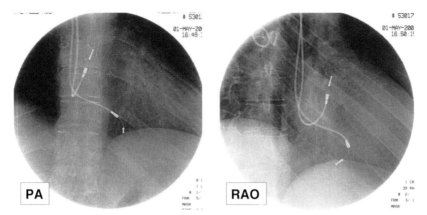

Figure 19.2 Ebstein's anomaly (pre valve). Two chest cine fluoroscopic views; Postero-anterior (PA) and right anterior oblique (RAO) showing dual chamber pacing in a patient with Ebstein's anomaly. The passive-fixation atrial lead lies in the atrial appendage. The passive-fixation right ventricular lead lies in the atrialized right ventricular cul de sac and the RAO view confirms that the tip is against the posterior wall. This pre valve position was confirmed by echocardiography and pacing thresholds were satisfactory although the patient was not pacemaker dependent.

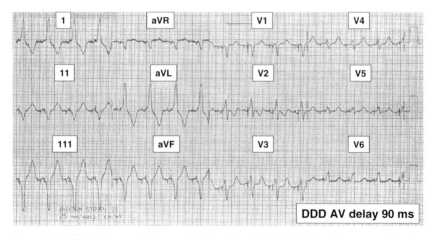

Figure 19.3 Ebstein's anomaly (pre valve). Resting 12-lead ECG from the same patient in Figure 19.2, demonstrating dual chamber pacing. Because of normal atrioventricular conduction, the atrioventricular delay was programmed to a short 90 ms to force ventricular pacing. The QRS configuration confirms right ventricular pacing with a superior or leftward axis.

Post-valve

Although technically difficult, it may be possible, particularly with milder forms of Ebstein's anomaly, to pass a transvenous ventricular lead through

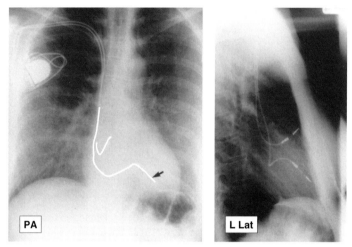

Figure 19.4 Ebstein's anomaly (post valve). Chest radiographs, postero-anterior (PA) and left lateral (L Lat), showing dual chamber pacing in a patient with Ebstein's anomaly. There is a passive-fixation lead in the right atrial appendage. The ventricular passive-fixation lead has been positioned at the apex of the true right ventricle beyond the malpositioned tricuspid valve. In the L Lat view the ventricular lead lies anterior. The lead position was confirmed by echocardiography.

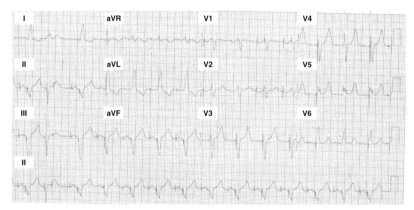

Figure 19.5 Ebstein's anomaly (post valve). Resting 12-lead ECG from the same patient in Figure 19.4, demonstrating dual chamber pacing. The pacemaker has been programmed DOO (to demonstrate consistent pacing). The features are identical to normal pacing from the apex of the right ventricle; left bundle branch block and left or superior axis.

the displaced tricuspid orifice and then angle the electrode towards the apex of the right ventricle (Figure 19.4). The ECG would again show a left bundle branch block appearance with a superior leftward axis (Figure 19.5). When attempting to position a lead post valve, an active-fixation screw-in

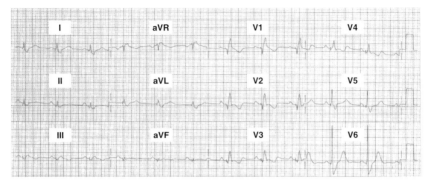

Figure 19.6 Ebstein's anomaly (cardiac vein). Resting 12-lead ECG demonstrating dual chamber pacing. The ventricular lead lies in the middle or a low lateral cardiac vein. There is atrial sensing and ventricular pacing with a right bundle branch block and a normal axis. This suggests left ventricular pacing from a site above the apex.

lead would be preferable, particularly if the lead can be anchored in the outflow tract. An active-fixation lead would also be preferable in the presence of tricuspid regurgitation. It is likely that the newly developed steerable catheter will be helpful in placing thin active-fixation leads (Figure 7.5).

Cardiac venous system

When the atrialized right ventricle is unsuitable or it is impossible to traverse the tricuspid orifice, ventricular pacing from the cardiac venous system may be an option. It may be possible to position a standard tined lead in one of the cardiac veins. The surface electrocardiogram shows left ventricular epicardial pacing with a right bundle branch block appearance and the axis will depend on where the lead lies. For instance, if the lead lies low in the heart such as in the middle or lateral cardiac vein, then there will be a leftward axis similar to pacing from the cardiac apex (Figure 19.6). In this position, the lateral chest x-ray helps confirm the cardiac venous pacing by demonstrating the characteristic posterior position of the ventricular lead tip (Figure 19.7). Generally leads placed inadvertently in this position provide stable pacing with low thresholds as long as the lead is gently wedged into a small venous tributary. It may be also possible to position a lead on the lateral left ventricular epicardial wall via the upper portion of the coronary sinus similar to the left ventricular leads of biventricular pacing. Although this would provide physiologic left ventricular pacing, nevertheless, in pacemaker-dependent patients, it would not be regarded as safe or desirable, because of the potential complications discussed earlier.

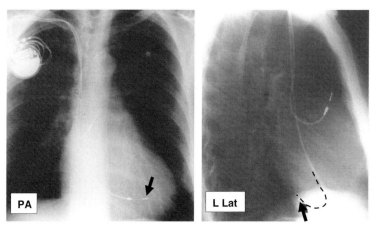

Figure 19.7 Ebstein's anomaly (cardiac vein). Chest radiographs, postero-anterior (PA) and left lateral (L Lat), showing dual chamber pacing in a patient with Ebstein's anomaly (same patient as in Figure 19.6). There is a passive-fixation lead in the right atrial appendage. The ventricular passive-fixation lead bypasses the malpositioned tricuspid valve by entering the coronary sinus and a cardiac vein which is most likely a low lateral cardiac vein (black arrow). In the L Lat view, the ventricular lead lies posterior which confirms that the lead is not in the right ventricle (black arrow). In this case the lead position was not confirmed by transthoracic echocardiography because of poor views. The patient refused a transesophageal echocardiograph.

Despite the variety of options available for transvenous lead placement, most patients have in the past received ventricular epicardial and epimyocardial leads [194]. This will be discussed further in the section on post-operative Ebstein's anomaly.

SECTION C

Previous corrective or palliative cardiac surgery

CHAPTER 20

D-Transposition of the great vessels

An infant born with dextro or D-transposition of the great vessels belongs to one of the cyanotic heart lesion categories and rarely survives the first year of life without surgical intervention [202]. The condition entails a normal embryogenic rightward cardiac loop, but failure of the great vessels to completely rotate. Therefore, the aorta arises from a normal right ventricle and, concomitantly, a pulmonary artery arises from the left ventricle. A venous-arterial circulation exists in parallel rather than in series with desaturated venous blood recirculating through the systemic circulation without first entering into the pulmonary circulation (Figure 20.1). Without some type of communication such as a patent ductus arteriosus or atrial or ventricular septal defects, infants succumb to cyanosis. The adult pacemaker and ICD implanter would therefore never encounter a patient with D-transposition of the great vessels who had not undergone corrective surgery.

Two physiologically related surgeries to correct the cyanosis are performed in the young: the Senning, and the more commonly used Mustard procedures; redirect venous blood by removal of the atrial septum followed by the insertion of an intra-atrial baffle (Figure 20.2). The baffle creates a physiologic blood flow redistribution in which the desaturated venous peripheral blood is directed to the mitral valve and left ventricle, which then exits to the transposed pulmonary artery. Saturated pulmonary venous blood is concomitantly directed to the right atrium, tricuspid valve, right ventricle and leaves the heart via the aorta. Often the infant may have first had an atrial septal defect created or a balloon atrial septostomy to acutely allow for mixing of arterial and venous blood to stabilize acid–base balance.

The Mustard procedure, which was first reported from Canada in 1964, uses atrial pericardium or synthetic materials as the intra-atrial baffle [203]. Soon after this atrial switch procedure was first described, there were a number of reports of early and late atrial arrhythmias and sudden

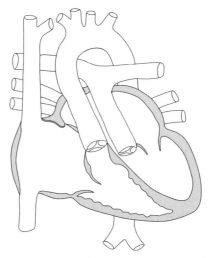

Figure 20.1 Schematic of transposition of the great vessels in the dextro or "D" position caused by a normal rightward looping of the embryogenic cardiac tube but an arrest of the normal rotation of the great vessels. As a result, there is atrio-ventricular concordance (atria and ventricles are normally joined), but ventriculo-arterial discordance (ventricles and great vessels are not correctly joined). As a consequence, the right-sided ventricle ejects desaturated venous blood back into the aorta and the left-sided ventricle ejects saturated pulmonary venous blood back to the pulmonary artery. Unless corrected, the condition is incompatible with life.

death, which diminished with a change in surgical technique particularly in regard to cannulation, suturing of the baffle and protection of the sinus node.

Although the survival rate for the Mustard procedure is generally regarded as good [204], long-term results continue to show a high incidence of sick sinus syndrome with brady and tachycardias and in particular junctional, rhythm and atrial tachyarrhythmias [205–208]. At least some of the sudden deaths were believed to be related to junctional rhythm, atrial flutter or complete heart block [209–212], particularly during exercise as a result of ventricular arrhythmias and therefore not prevented by cardiac pacing [213].

The Senning operation for correction of D-transposition of the great vessels was described before the Mustard procedure [214]. In this operation, the systemic and pulmonary venous return are rerouted using flaps of the atrial septum and right atrial free wall. Although no foreign material is used, the early results were not particularly good and consequently very few reports of this operation were published after the introduction of the Mustard procedure [215, 216]. Because of the extensive atrial surgery

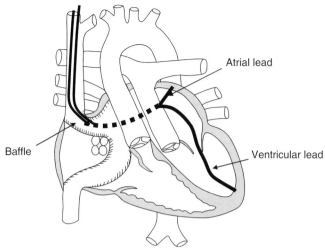

Figure 20.2 D-transposition of the great vessels and lead placement. Schematic of the intra-atrial baffle associated with the Mustard and Senning procedures. After removal of the inter-atrial septum, the baffle allows desaturated vena caval venous blood to be directed to the left atrium and ventricle which then permits flow into the pulmonary artery. Saturated pulmonary venous return is directed to the right atrium, right ventricle and aorta. Atrial and ventricular pacing leads have been positioned. Both pass behind the baffle at the junction of the right atrium with the superior vena cava (broken line). The atrial lead must then be positioned on the roof of the left atrium, whereas the ventricular lead traverses the mitral valve to the lateral wall of the left ventricle.

required, it is not surprising that sinus node damage was frequent and that there was a high incidence of atrial arrhythmias and late mortality, comparable to the Mustard procedure [217].

At the present time, there still exists a significant subset of adult patients who have undergone a palliative Mustard or Senning procedure. Some of these patients, who reach adulthood had associated ventricular septal defects and developed irreversible pulmonary hypertension. The atrial baffle improves mixing and increases systemic saturations to 70–85%. However, the ventricular defect remains open. Such patients are typically treated with aspirin. If pacing is required, addition of a transvenous pacing system will require coumadin therapy to prevent thromboembolic events. If ventricular pacing is necessary, the presence of a persistent ventricular septal defect will limit lead placement. For instance left ventricular septal or outflow tract pacing, which may be desirable to preserve right ventricular function, will not be possible.

As the young recipients of either procedure entered adulthood, more and more required cardiac pacing to alleviate the symptoms of

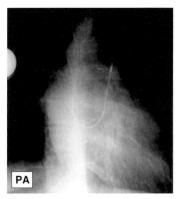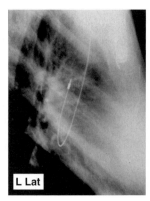

Figure 20.3 Mustard procedure for D-transposition of the great vessels. Chest radiographs, postero-anterior (PA) and left lateral (L Lat), showing left atrial pacing in a patient with the Mustard procedure. In the PA view an active-fixation lead has been passed from the right subclavicular region to the superior vena cava and the stub of the right atrium. It then proceeds behind the baffle into the anatomical left atrium, where it is attached to the roof. In the L Lat view, the lead lies posterior which is very different to the traditional right atrial appendage position. In this case, intermittent left phrenic nerve stimulation occurred.

bradyarrhythmias and tachyarrhythmias. With the gradual introduction of the technically demanding but more physiologic, great vessel or arterial switch procedure originally described by Dr Jatene in the late 1970s [218], the atrial baffle procedures were slowly abandoned. Because the Jatene or arterial switch operation does not involve the atria, sinus node dysfunction does not usually occur. However, the surgery does involve excision and reimplantation of coronary arteries. Therefore, there is some risk to sinus or AV nodal arteries and on occasion a pacemaker or ICD may be required. If so, then it should be regarded as a routine procedure, with normal ventricular orientation and configuration. However, in those patients who first underwent a palliative balloon atrial septostomy to stabilize acid-base balance prior to definitive cardiac repair, an atrial defect patch may have been used to close the defect. The presence of such material may complicate atrial lead insertion, especially if Bachmann's bundle pacing is anticipated.

To the uninitiated implanter, insertion of a pacemaker or ICD in a patient with D-transposition of the great vessels corrected with either the Senning or Mustard procedures, conjures up a frightening scenario. Once the anatomy is understood, the actual implantation is very straightforward. However, for a successful outcome, a number of factors must be considered.

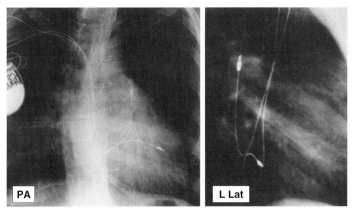

Figure 20.4 Mustard procedure for transposition of the great vessels. Chest radiographs, postero-anterior (PA) and left lateral (L Lat), showing dual chamber pacing in a patient with the Mustard procedure. In the PA view, an active-fixation lead is attached to the roof of the left atrium. The active-fixation ventricular lead passes behind the baffle and through the anatomical mitral valve into the body of the left ventricle and is attached to the lateral wall. In the L Lat view, both leads lie posterior. In this case, both leads caused left phrenic nerve stimulation with high voltage output pacing.

Provided the pathway is clear, the atrial lead progresses through the superior vena cava and the stub of the right atrium and proceeds behind the baffle into the anatomical left atrium (Figures 20.2–20.4). A straight steroid-eluting screw-in lead with a curved stylet should be used and the lead positioned as medial (right) as possible to prevent phrenic nerve stimulation, which unfortunately is a common post implant complication [209,219]. In this situation, the steerable stylet (Locator® Model 4036, St Jude Medical, Minneapolis, Mn.) is extremely useful (Figure 7.1). The lead can be very easily placed into the anatomic left atrium using a standard curved stylet and then positioned medially on the roof, well away from the phrenic nerve, using the maximum curve of the Locator®. Because of the sharp curve required, the lead may not be adequately secured to the left atrial wall. Withdrawing the Locator® stylet with a modest curve still present will provide enough stress on the distal end to dislodge the lead if it isn't adequately secured (Figures 20.5, 20.6). The recent introduction of the steerable catheter delivery system (Figure 7.5) has also facilitated lead implant in the left atrium by permitting a more acute angle to reach the roof of the left atrium (Figure 20.7).

One of the major issues with pacemaker or ICD implantation is the presence of venous or baffle stenosis hindering the transvenous pathway to the left ventricle [220, 221]. Obstruction to the intra-atrial baffle,

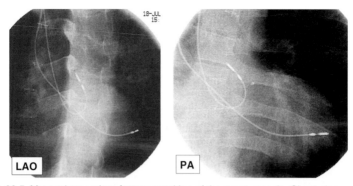

Figure 20.5 Mustard procedure for transposition of the great vessels. Chest cine fluoroscopic 40° left anterior oblique (LAO) and postero-anterior (PA) views, showing dual chamber pacing in a patient with the Mustard procedure. In both views, the upper active-fixation lead is attached to the roof of the left atrium, but unlike in Figures 20.3 and 20.4, the attachment is arched more medial, well away from the left phrenic nerve. The left ventricular lead is attached to the body of the chamber and testing revealed no diaphragmatic stimulation with both leads.

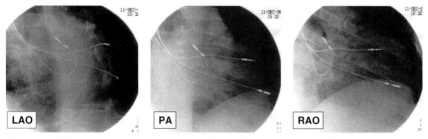

Figure 20.6 Mustard procedure for transposition of the great vessels. Chest cine fluoroscopic 28° left anterior oblique (LAO), postero-anterior (PA) and 28° right anterior oblique (RAO) views, showing dual chamber pacing in a patient with the Mustard procedure. In all views, the upper active-fixation lead is attached to the roof of the left atrium, but unlike in Figures 20.3 and 20.4, the attachment is arched more medial, well away from the left phrenic nerve. There are two active-fixation leads in the left ventricular chamber. The lower one is not functioning.

typically at the superior vena cava junction due to patient growth and angulation, can occur in about 22% of patients, many years after the Mustard or Senning procedures [222]. Unfortunately, such obstructions may not be clinically evident as the azygous vein often serves to decompress the stenosis by permitting venous runoff to the inferior vena caval system. The more posterior location of the azygous vein and vena cava also preclude effective echocardiographic/Doppler evaluations. When

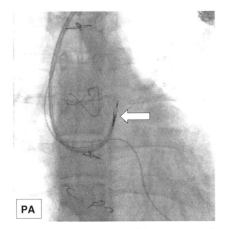

Figure 20.7 Mustard procedure for transposition of the great vessels. Chest cine fluoroscopic, postero-anterior (PA) view demonstrating the use of the SelectSite™ catheter delivery system through the superior vena cava baffle, facilitating lead placement at the medial location on the roof of the venous left atrium. The acute curvature of the delivery catheter allows selective lead placement in previously technically difficult to reach locations.

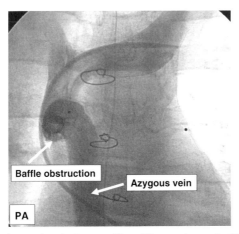

Figure 20.8 Mustard procedure for transposition of the great vessels. Chest cine fluoroscopic, postero-anterior (PA) view of a superior vena caval venogram illustrating a dilated posterior directed azygous vein associated with superior vena cava baffle obstruction. Venous blood flow eventually communicates with the inferior vena cava.

such a situation is suspected, investigations such as magnetic resonance imaging, computerized tomographic scans or venograms are required to delineate the venous anatomy prior to attempted pacemaker implant (Figure 20.8).

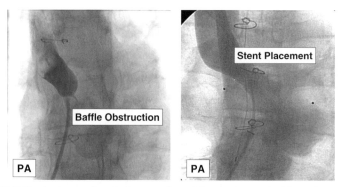

Figure 20.9 Mustard procedure for transposition of the great vessels. Chest cine fluoroscopic, postero-anterior (PA) views of a superior vena caval venogram. *Left:* Baffle obstruction at the junction of the baffle with the right atrium and superior vena cava. *Right:* Stent placement with wide opening of the baffle. Patient growth and vena caval-baffle angulation typically is responsible for such obstructions.

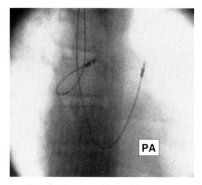

Figure 20.10 Mustard procedure for transposition of the great vessels. Chest cine fluoroscopic, postero-anterior (PA) view, showing bipolar atrial pacing in a patient with the Mustard procedure from an era before bipolar leads were available. One lead (cathode) is in the left atrium and the other (anode) is attached to baffle material as it it was not possible to attach it to the stump of the right atrium. The anode lead would not pace the atrium, but the lead combination allowed satisfactory long-term bipolar atrial pacing.

Once identified vascular stents can be effectively used to open the obstructed baffle regions followed by pacing lead implant (Figure 20.9). However, due to continued lead-stent neo-intimal interactions following implant, vessel restenosis may reoccur necessitating continued close follow-up care [64]. In a patient with sick sinus syndrome and baffle stenosis, it may still be possible to position an atrial lead into a stub of right atrial appendage close to where it attaches to the baffle (Figure 20.10) [223]. On intraoperative testing, atrial pacing may not be possible or a very high

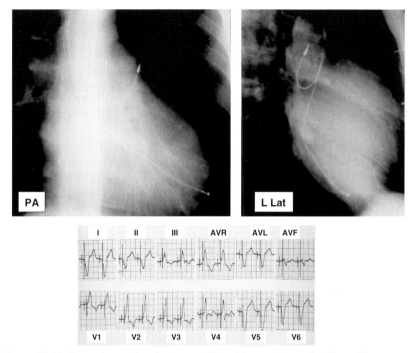

Figure 20.11 Mustard procedure for transposition of the great vessels. *Above:* Chest radiographs, postero-anterior (PA) and left lateral (L Lat), showing dual chamber pacing in a patient with the Mustard procedure. In the PA view, active-fixation leads are attached to the roof of the left atrium and lateral wall of the left ventricle. In the L Lat view, both leads lie posterior. *Below:* Resting 12-lead ECG from the same patient demonstrating dual chamber pacing with a right bundle branch block indicating left ventricular pacing. There is a right axis deviation suggesting that the lead is not at the apex of the left ventricle, but rather higher up in the body of the chamber.

stimulation threshold is recorded. In this situation the lead is actually in contact with the baffle material and must be repositioned.

For ventricular pacing, the lead must be passed to the left atrium and then via the anatomical mitral valve to the left ventricle where it is positioned in the body of the chamber [224]. The major concern once again is phrenic nerve stimulation which must be tested using 10 volts output from the pacing system analyser.

The electrocardiograph of dual chamber pacing in patients with the Mustard or Senning procedure for transposition of the great vessels shows classical left ventricular pacing with dominant R waves from V1 to V4 (Figure 20.11). The axis is, however, dependent on the position of the lead in the left ventricle. The higher the lead in the chamber, the more prominent the R wave in lead III (Figures 20.12, 20.13).

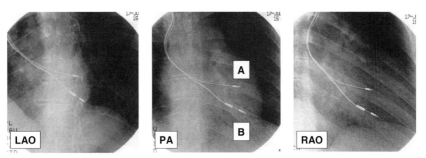

Figure 20.12 Mustard procedure for transposition of the great vessels. Chest cine fluoroscopic 40° left anterior oblique (LAO), postero-anterior (PA) and 26° right anterior oblique (RAO) views, showing dual site left ventricular pacing in a patient with the Mustard procedure. The upper lead (unipolar) lies just under the mitral valve whereas the lower lead lies in the body of the chamber.

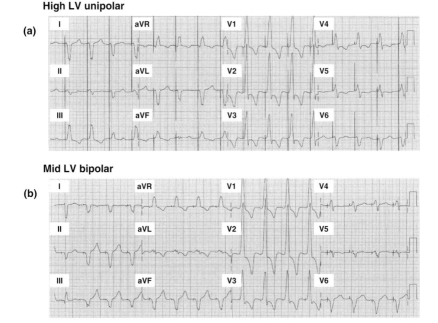

Figure 20.13 Mustard procedure for transposition of the great vessels. Two resting 12-lead ECGs of the single chamber pacing system shown in Figure 20.12 demonstrating left ventricular (LV) pacing. The upper ECG shows unipolar pacing from the lead just below the mitral valve and the lower is bipolar pacing from the mid left ventricle. Unlike right ventricular pacing, there is little difference in the ECGs from the two sites.

CHAPTER 21

Septal defects including tetralogy of fallot

It has been well known since the 1950s that surgery for congenital heart disease and in particular ventricular septal defects may acutely result in atrioventricular block requiring temporary and occasionally permanent pacing. This was the result of trauma and edema to the atrioventricular node, His bundle and more distal conducting pathways. The block probably resulted from septal sutures [225, 226] and often settled during the early post operative phase. With increasing knowledge of the aberrant conduction tissue pathways, particularly with ventricular septal defects, the incidence of these problems diminished. However, post operatively the patients frequently demonstrated ECG evidence of conduction tissue damage, which was confirmed with electrophysiology studies [227]. Although often regarded as benign [228, 229], cases of symptomatic complete heart block and sudden death were reported years later, similar to the sick sinus syndrome scenario seen with D-transposition of the great vessels and the Mustard procedure [230, 231].

In patients with a single surgical repair such as a ventricular septal defect, the cause could be attributed to the septal sutures, whereas with more complex surgery as with tetralogy of Fallot, the exact identification of the cause is more complex [225]. For obvious reasons, the more distal the conduction tissue damage, the less likely the surgery will result in complete heart block. This fact may also be of significance with the onset of complete heart block, years later [225]. Of particular importance is that transient complete heart block at the time of surgery in association with ongoing bifascicular block, is a more powerful predictor for developing either late complete heart block or sudden death, than either bifascicular block or transient heart block alone [225, 232]. Similarly, the progression of a bundle branch block to trifascicular block also carries a high risk of sudden death [233].

Not all ventricular septal defects require surgery. Thus the implanter may encounter a patient with a small ventricular septal defect (Maladie de Roger) in adulthood who requires a ventricular pacing lead (Figure 21.1).

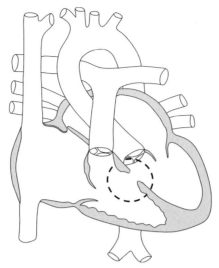

Figure 21.1 Schematic sketch of a ventricular septal defect. The most common site as shown (broken circle) is the Perimembranous defect (type 2). Other septal defect locations include Supracristal (type 1), Inflow or AV Canal (type 3) and Muscular (type 4).

As with the atrial septal defect, care must be taken to ensure that the lead is not inadvertently placed in the left ventricle. Obviously, the same principles of management as with an atrial septal defect apply (Chapter 16).

Care must also be taken if the ventricular lead is to be positioned in the right ventricular outflow tract as areas of scarring are to be avoided. Consideration should be given to device closure prior to positioning the ventricular lead (Figure 21.2). If the septal defect remains open after lead insertion anticoagulation with coumadin should be considered.

An important fact to remember when investigating a patient who has had a ventriculotomy earlier in life is the likely presence of a right bundle branch block configuration. The presence of certain congenital defects, such as an atrioventricular septal defect, inherently causes a QRS left axis shift and AV node conduction delay. An intracardiac electrophysiology study may also demonstrate prolonged H-V intervals. However, such patients may not have progressive fascicular conduction disease and may not truly be candidates for permanent pacing based on those criteria alone. As in any evaluation, clinical presentation is mandatory.

Not surprisingly, there is also an increased incidence of bradycardia-tachycardia syndromes following atrial septal defect surgery. This may be related to the surgery on the septum or the surgical incisions in the free wall or appendage [234].

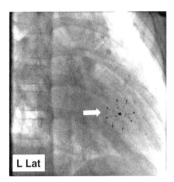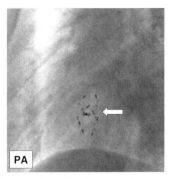

Figure 21.2 Ventricular septal defect device closure. Chest cine fluoroscopic postero-anterior (PA) and left lateral (L Lat) views, of a star shaped Cardioseal® device (NMT Medical, Boston, MA, USA) (white arrows) inserted into a mid-muscular located ventricular septal defect. The device size and location may proclude effective septal tract lead placement.

Since the anatomic pathways to the right atrium and ventricle are normal, there should be no surprises when implanting a transvenous cardiac pacemaker in a patient who has had an atrial or ventricular septal defect closed. However, the presence of enlarged and potentially scared right sided chambers may make the procedure long, tedious, and more likely to result in lead dislodgement. Even if the implanting physician's preferred leads are tined, it is prudent to choose from the outset, active fixation leads as the traditional sites may not be suitable. Examples of difficult lead implants due to interference from ventricular patch material are demonstrated with an inflow tract attachment in Figure 21.3 and a high outflow tract attachment in Figure 21.4.

Patients with repaired complete atrioventricular septal defect (endocardial cushion defect) may be particularly difficult cases for ventricular lead placement. There is often extensive septal synthetic patch material limiting the sites for successful pacing. The repaired tricuspid valves of such patients may be regurgitant making lead placement difficult. In such cases where the patient may become pacemaker-dependent, the "belt and braces" technique discussed in Chapter 8 should be considered [65].

Another complicating problem may occur with the recent introduction of interventional devices to close ventricular septal defects. The patients will not have a sternal or thoracotomy scar and thus the significance of the closure device may be missed. For those implanters who use the right ventricular outflow tract there may be significant technical difficulties in effective septal lead placement (Figure 21.2)

The tetralogy of Fallot, first described by Fallot in 1888, is one of the most common congenital heart defects causing cyanosis. The

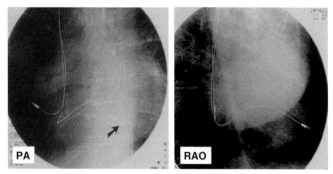

Figure 21.3 Ventricular septal defect repair. Chest cine fluoroscopic postero-anterior (PA) and right anterior oblique (RAO) views, showing an implanted dual chamber lead system in a patient following repair of a large ventricular septal defect. The active-fixation right atrial lead is on the low antero-lateral wall and the active-fixation right ventricular lead is in the inflow tract of a large right ventricular chamber (black arrow). Attempts to pass the ventricular lead toward the apex resulted in high stimulation thresholds.

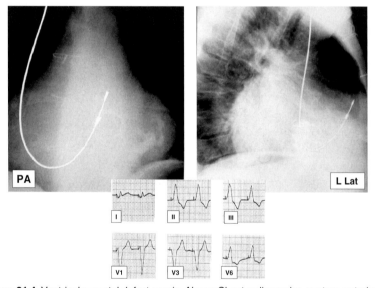

Figure 21.4 Ventricular septal defect repair. *Above:* Chest radiographs, postero-anterior (PA) and left lateral (L Lat), showing an implanted ventricular lead in a patient following repair of a very large ventricular septal defect and replacement of the mitral valve. The active-fixation lead has been positioned high in the right ventricular outflow tract. *Below:* Resting 6-lead ECG, demonstrating the typical appearance of ventricular pacing from that site (see Figure 5.2).

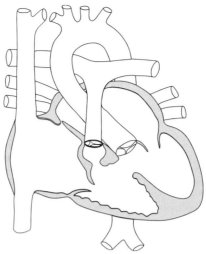

Figure 21.5 Schematic sketch of tetralogy of Fallot. The four basic components; right ventricular outflow obstruction, ventricular septal defect, aorta "overriding" the VSD and right ventricular hypertrophy are illustrated. Typically the pulmonary obstruction is sub-valvular in the outflow muscle, although associated pulmonary valve stenosis can occur. In addition to the VSD closure, surgical repair may involve a trans-annular patch placed across the pulmonary valve which may enlarge the outflow tract but exacerbate pulmonary valve insufficiency.

anatomico-pathologic tetralogy consists of an antero-cephalad deviation of the infundibular right ventricular outflow tract with resultant obstruction, a ventricular septal defect, the rightward displacement of the aorta over the ventricular septal defect, and right ventricular hypertrophy (Figure 21.5) [235]. The addition of an atrial septal defect creates a pentalogy of Fallot. An atrial septal defect or patent foramen ovale may be present in 82% and a left superior vena cava draining to the coronary sinus in 11% of patients [236]. Physiologically-related congenital heart conditions include double outlet right ventricle and pulmonary atresia.

Typically, the patient with tetralogy of Fallot, presenting for pacemaker or ICD implant, will have had a preliminary systemic to pulmonary artery anastomosis to improve saturation as an infant (Blalock-Taussig, Waterston, Potts, Cooley or central graft) followed by the more definitive intracardiac repair later in life. If the subclavian artery was used, there may be subsequent loss of the pulse on that respective arm. Surgical repair typically includes patch closure of septal defects with opening of the narrowed right ventricular infundibulum by placement of a synthetic or pericardial patch up to or across the pulmonary valve annulus. Most patients will exhibit at least moderate pulmonary valve insufficiency which

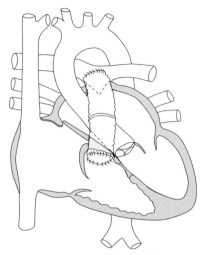

Figure 21.6 Schematic sketch of repair of tetralogy of Fallot. Among patients with nearly complete outflow tract atresia, surgical repair may involve a valved or non-valved conduit (Rastelli procedure) to effectively create a jump graft from the right ventricle to pulmonary artery.

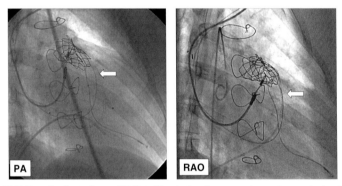

Figure 21.7 Repair of tetralogy of Fallot. Chest cine fluoroscopic postero-anterior (PA) and right anterior oblique (RAO) views of a patient following Rastelli repair of a tetralogy of Fallot. A prior conduit stenosis has been relieved by stent placement. There is a dual chamber lead system implanted with prolapse of the body of the tined ventricular lead into a valveless conduit (arrows) as result of free-regurgitant flow. This situation would make future lead extraction potentially more challenging. An active-fixation atrial lead is in the atrial appendage.

causes right ventricular dilatation and can complicate ventricular lead placement. In instances of more severe right ventricular outflow obstruction or valve atresia, a valve or valveless conduit (Rastelli) is attached from the right ventricular free wall, extending into the main pulmonary artery (Figure 21.6).

As expected, following the complicated repair of a tetralogy of Fallot, the heart will exhibit an extensive amount of ventricular fibrosis which can complicate pacemaker or ICD implantation. In such patients, the right ventricular apex, free wall and outflow regions may consist of synthetic material which will limit effective lead insertion. In addition, free pulmonary insufficiency with associated blood flow turbulence may cause excessive lead movement with the potential for excursion into the outflow tract (Figure 21.7). Elevated post-implant pacing thresholds may be anticipated as well as difficulty during lead extraction.

The potential for ventricular arrhythmias and sudden death has been reported as high as 38% among patients with premature ventricular complexes and elevated ventricular pressures due to recurrent outflow tract obstruction [237]. Therefore determination of ventricular pressures prior to pacemaker implantation may help in determining if the patient is a candidate for concomitant interventional balloon angioplasty or additional surgical relief of any residual outflow tract obstruction. Such a patient being considered for a pacemaker may in fact benefit from an ICD.

CHAPTER 22

Repaired Ebstein's anomaly

Conduction tissue disease is one of the features of Ebstein's anomaly, which usually denotes a more severe form of the syndrome and consequently such patients may require tricuspid valve reconstructive surgery or replacement [194]. If at open heart surgery, an annuloplasty has been performed, pacing or ICD leads can still be inserted into the right ventricle (Figure 22.1) [39]. However, once a mechanical prosthetic valve has been implanted, a transvenous lead cannot be positioned in the ventricle via the valve orifice. Consideration should, therefore, be given to the implantation of a ventricular lead at the time of the original surgery. As described earlier, the lead can be positioned in the ventricle, via the atrium and the sewing ring of the prosthetic tricuspid valve will then cover the lead as it traverses the annulus (Figure 4.3). This lead can be tunneled to the anterior abdominal wall or subclavicular area and if not used immediately can be capped and buried. Such a procedure would be potentially very helpful, if there is evidence of sick sinus syndrome or atrioventricular block which may progress in the future.

Another situation in Ebstein's anomaly that may require cardiac pacing in the future is the propensity for atrial fibrillation. In the presence of a large atrium resultant from long-standing tricuspid regurgitation, atrial fibrillation may be present preoperatively or may occur post-operatively. A pacemaker may be indicated either at surgery or sometime after it for a slow ventricular response, inappropriate pauses or the need to consider His bundle ablation.

If a ventricular lead is required in the presence of a mechanical tricuspid valve prosthesis, an endocardial lead can still be passed via the transvenous route to the coronary sinus and placed in a cardiac vein on the epicardial surface [68–74]. However, as discussed in chapter 1, post operatively the coronary sinus may not drain directly into the right atrium. The surgeon, in order to protect the conducting system may position the prosthetic tricuspid valve, so that the coronary sinus lies on the ventricular side of the

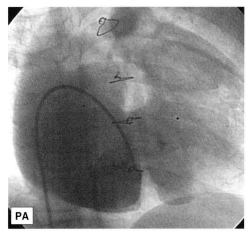

Figure 22.1 Ebstein's anomaly. Chest cine fluoroscopic postero-anterior (PA) view of a right ventriculogram demonstrating the relatively narrow effective tricuspid valve orifice associated with severe insufficiency and dilatation of the right atrium in a postoperative patient with Ebstein's anomaly.

valve. The surgical notes should, therefore, be reviewed pre implant and if necessary attempts made to visualize the ostium of the coronary sinus before embarking on the pacemaker implantation.

In most cases where the tricuspid valve has been replaced, an epicardial pacing system will be used. The lead must be attached to the epimyocardial ventricular wall in an area scarred from previous surgery. An open heart, transatrial approach to position an active-fixation lead in the right ventricular outflow tract has also been described in an Ebstein's anomaly patient with a tricuspid annuloplasty [39].

SECTION D

No venous access to ventricle

CHAPTER 23

Univentricular heart

The univentricular heart represents a broad spectrum of congenital abnormalities of the heart and great vessels, where the common abnormality is a single ventricle. This concept is typically associated with any of six possible anatomical variations of tricuspid atresia, most of which are associated with a non-existant or rudimentary venous ventricle (Figure 23.1).

The Fontan procedure, to separate and redirect venous blood flow, presents the most challenging pacing options for the adult with congenital

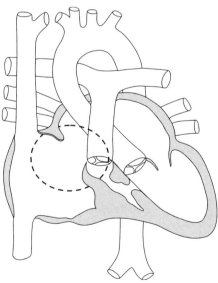

Figure 23.1 Schematic of tricuspid atresia (univentricular heart) (type 1B). The right ventricle and outflow pulmonary artery are rudimentary and effectively non-existent. In this defect, survival depends on an effective atrial septal communication (broken ring).

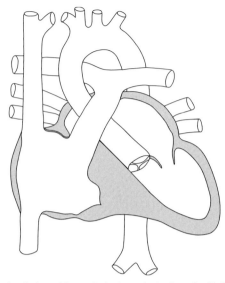

Figure 23.2 Schematic of tricuspid atresia (univentricular heart) with Fontan repair. In the more classic "Fontan" surgical repair, the atrial septal defect is closed and a direct right atrial (RA) - pulmonary artery (PA) anastomosis created. The ultimately elevated atrial pressures (often in the range of 20mmHg) eventually cause severe atrial dilatation and wall thickening. As expected, sinus node dysfunction and atrial arrhythmias are common.

heart disease. The operation and its many modifications is performed in up to four surgical procedures in order to separate the systemic and pulmonary circulations. This is accomplished by either a direct anastomosis of the right atrium to the pulmonary artery (Figure 23.2) or any variations of anastomoses involving the superior and inferior venae cavae to the pulmonary artery using an intra-atrial tunnel or extra-cardiac conduit. These latter techniques are referred to as *total cavopulmonary connection*. As might be expected, a lateral tunnel or external conduit repair may preclude use of transvenous atrial pacing as the vena cava may no longer communicate with the atrial chamber. Thus, it is essential that the operation notes be reviewed before consideration of a transvenous atrial lead placement.

Early reported procedures, describe a direct connection between the right atrium and the pulmonary artery causing extensive dilatation and damage to the right atrium (Figure 23.3) [238]. The right atrioventricular (tricuspid) valve orifice and pulmonary valve orifice, if present, were closed denying access by the transvenous route to the univentricular chamber. Because of the extensive and cumulative atrial damage with each operation, there is a high incidence of postoperative arrhythmias with primarily loss of sinus rhythm [239–243]. Thus, it is not unusual for patients who have undergone the Fontan procedure in childhood to present for cardiac

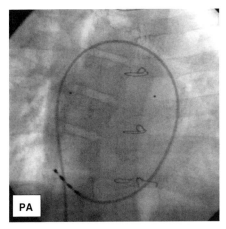

Figure 23.3 Tricuspid atresia (univentricular heart). Chest cine fluoroscopic postero-anterior (PA) view demonstrating a very dilated right atrium following a classic Fontan procedure. The 6Fr quadripolar pacing catheter demarcates the extent of the atrial dimensions.

pacing as a teenager or adult with atrial bradyarrhythmias and intact atrioventricular conduction [238].

The conventional method of atrial pacing following the Fontan procedure is right atrial epimyocardial [244]. However, because of multiple previous cardiac operations and atrial scarring, extensive dissection is required to obtain satisfactory pacing and sensing and the left atrium has been suggested as an alternative site [245, 246]. Despite the perceived difficulties, good results have been documented using the epicardial approach [247]. Transmural placement of the lead into the right atrium at thoracotomy has also been reported [248].

If there is a venous passageway to the right atrium, traditional single chamber transvenous atrial pacing can be successfully performed [63, 238, 244, 249, 250] Because of the theoretical risk of obstructing venous flow into the pulmonary artery, small diameter leads are recommended and in particular, the SelectSecure® lead inserted with a steerable catheter, the SelectSite® (Figure 7.5) [63]. In such situations, the question arises as to the value of long-term oral anticoagulants such as coumadin. Seeing that there is such a high incidence of atrial tachyarrhythmias such as atrial flutter as well, it seems prudent to make such a recommendation.

Atrioventricular block tends to occur following the Fontan procedure in older children or young adults undergoing the surgery [63, 250]. Because, there is no connection to the single ventricle, ventricular pacing cannot be accomplished theoretically by the transvenous route. Consequently, the ventricular lead should must be positioned on the epimyocardial surface [247]. Because of the difficulties obtaining satisfactory long-term atrial

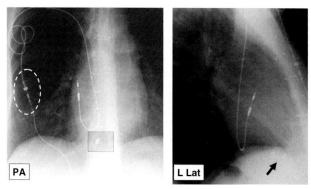

Figure 23.4 Tricuspid atresia (univentricular heart). Chest radiographs, postero-anterior (PA) and left lateral (L Lat), showing dual chamber pacing in a patient with a univentricular heart who had previously undergone a Fontan procedure. In the PA view, a transvenous active-fixation lead is attached to the antero-lateral right atrial wall. This lead is then brought down to the anterior abdominal wall using a connector (white oval) buried behind the breast. For ventricular pacing, two screw-in epimyocardial leads are attached to the lowermost portion of the single ventricle. The two epimyocardial leads are on top of each other in the PA view which has been highlighted with a box. In the L Lat view, a black arrow points to the two epimyocardial leads, one behind the other.

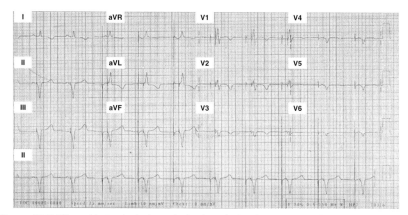

Figure 23.5 Tricuspid atresia (univentricular heart). Resting 12-lead ECG from the same patient in Figure 23.4, demonstrating dual chamber pacing. There is both sensing and pacing in the atrium. Ventricular pacing demonstrates a right bundle branch block configuration and a left axis deviation suggesting left ventricular pacing from the apical region. The QRS complexes probably show fusion.

pacing, it is best where possible to perform dual chamber pacing using a two stage hybrid procedure if possible. The atrial lead can be implanted via the transvenous route. Following the second stage attachment of the epicardial/epimyocardial lead the pulse generator can be inserted in the subclavicular fossa or the atrial lead can be extended and brought down to the anterior abdominal wall. The pulse generator can then be attached in the abdomen (Figure 23.4). In this situation, the ventricular lead is attached anatomically and physiologically to the left ventricle giving rise to a right bundle branch block appearance on the ECG (Figure 23.5).

Despite the assumed lack of ventricular access, there have been cases of successful transvenously positioning of ventricular leads in patients having undergone a Fontan procedure. This can been achieved by the coronary sinus route if accessible [251] puncturing the dacron graft covering the tricuspid orifice [252] or puncturing the intra-atrial tunnel with a trans-septal needle [63, 253]. There have been successful cases of transvenous lead positioning in patients with univentricular hearts, who have not had the Fontan procedure [241, 250, 254].

Because of the high incidence of atrial tachyarrhythmias it is worth considering implanting a pulse generator with antitachycardia capabilities. This should include atrial overdrive pacing and maybe atrial reversion therapies.

Concluding remarks

As children born with congenital heart disease continue to age, physicians caring for adults will be exposed to this increasing population of patients. At the time of this publication, only the "tip of the iceberg" is visible. With an incidence of approximately 1% of live births and ever-improving surgical and device technologies, congenital heart patients will continue to survive to adulthood in increasing numbers. Based on the US National Center for Health Statistics, by 2020 the number of children in the United States born with congenital heart disease in 1990 alone will approximate 760,000 individuals [255]. Other countries may expect similar numbers.

The authors of this text have attempted to provide the reader with a glimpse into some of the technical challenges associated with pacemaker and ICD device implantation in these patients. By no means is this text inclusive of all congenital heart defects and all problems and pitfalls. As newer technologies evolve, the implanting physician will continue to face new and diverse challenges and will always require ingenuity and tricks to overcome them.

References

1 Giudici MC. Experience with a cosmetic approach to device implantation. *PACE* 2001; **24**: 1679–1680.

2 Mond HG. *The Cardiac Pacemaker. Function and Malfunction*. Harcourt Brace Jovanovich, New York 1983: 199.

3 Jacobs DM, Fink AS, Miller RP et al. Anatomical and Morphologic evaluation of pacemaker lead compression. *PACE* 1993; **16**: 434–444.

4 Ong LS, Barold S, Lederman M et al. Cephalic vein guide technique for implantation of permanent pacemakers. *Am Heart J* 1987; **114**: 753–756.

5 Rao G. Letter to the Editor. *PACE* 1981; **4**: 39.

6 Camous JP, Raybaud F, Lesto I et al. Introduction of permanent cardiac stimulation/defibrillation leads via the retro-pectoral veins. *PACE* 2005; **28**: 324–325.

7 Arnold AG. Permanent cardiac pacing using anterior pectoral veins. *Br Heart J* 1980; **43**: 321–323.

8 Gosalbez F, Cofino J, Llorente A et al. Retroclavicular route for electrode placement in endocardial pacemakers. *Chest* 1976; **70**: 679–683.

9 Belott PH. Blind axillary venous access. *PACE* 1999; **22**: 1085–1089.

10 Burri H, Sunthorn H, Dorsaz PA et al. Prospective study of axillary vein puncture with or without contrast venography for pacemaker and defibrillator lead implantation. *PACE* 2005; **28**: S280–S283.

11 Byrd CL. Clinical experience with the extrathoracic introducer insertion technique. *PACE* 1993; **16**: 1781–1784.

12 Belott PH, Reynolds DW. Permanent pacemaker and implantable cardioverter-defibrillator implantation. In: Ellenbogen, Kay, Wilkoff, eds. *Clinical Cardiac Pacing and Defibrillation*, 2nd edn. WB Saunders Co. Philadelphia 2000: 573–644.

13 Mond HG. *The Cardiac Pacemaker. Function and Malfunction*. Harcourt Brace Jovanovich, New York 1983: 201.

14 Ellestad MH, French J. Iliac vein approach to permanent pacemaker implantation. *PACE* 1989; **12**: 1030–1033.

15 Antonelli D, Freeberg NA, Rosenfeld T. Transiliac vein approach to a rate-responsive permanent pacemaker implantation. *PACE* 1993; **16**: 1751–1752.

16 Barakat K, Hill J, Kelly P. Permanent transfemoral pacemaker implantation is the technique of choice for patients in whom the super vena cava is inaccessible. *PACE* 2000; **23**: 446–449.

17 Giudici MC, Paul DL, Meierbachtol CJ. Active-can implantable cardioverter-defibrillator placement from a femoral approach. *PACE* 2003; **26**: 1297–1298.

18 Garcia Guerrero JJ, De La Concha Castaneda JF, Mora GF et al. Permanent trans-femoral pacemaker: A single-center series performed with an easier and safer surgical technique. *PACE* 2005; **28**: 675–679.

19 Fishberger SB, Camunas J, Rodriguez-Fernandez H et al. Permanent pacemaker lead implantation via the transhepatic route. *PACE* 1996; **19**: 1124–1125.

20 West JNW, Shearmann CP, Gammage MD. Permanent pacemaker positioning via the inferior vena cava in a case of single ventricle with loss of right atrial-vena cava continuity. *PACE* 1993; **16**: 1753–1755.

21 Bayliss CE, Beanlands DS, Baird RJ. The pacemaker-twiddlers syndrome: A new complication of implantable transvenous pacemakers. *Can Med Assoc J* 1968; **99**: 371–373.

22 Ventri EP, Mower MM, Reid PR. Twiddler's syndrome. A new twist. *PACE* 1984; **7**: 1004–1009.

23 Anderson MH, Nathan AW. Ventricular pacing from the atrial channel of a VDD pacemaker: A consequence of pacemaker twiddling? *PACE* 1990; **13**: 1567–1570.

24 Roberts JS, Wenger NK. Pacemaker twiddler's syndrome. *Am J Cardiol* 1989; **63**: 1013–1016.

25 Robinson LA, Windle JR. Defibrillator twiddler's syndrome. *Ann Thorac Surg* 1994; **58**: 247–249.

26 Beauregard LM, Russo AM, Heim J et al. Twiddler's syndrome complicating automatic defibrillator function. *PACE* 1995; **18**: 735–737.

27 Mehta D, Lipsius M, Suri RS et al. Twiddler's syndrome with the implantable cardioverter-defibrillator. *Am Heart J* 1992; **123**: 1079–1082.

28 Higgins SL, Suh BD, Stein JB et al. Recurrent twiddler's syndrome in a nonthora-cotomy ICD system despite a Dacron pouch. *PACE* 1998; **21**: 130–133.

29 Bohm A, Komaromy K, Pinter A et al. Pacemaker lead fracture due to twiddler's syndrome. *PACE* 1998; **21**: 1162–1163.

30 Saliba BC, Ghantous AE, Schoenfeld MH et al. Twiddler's syndrome with trans-venous defibrillators in the pectoral region. *PACE* 1999; **22**: 1419–1421.

31 Kistler P, Eizenberg N, Fynn SP et al. The subpectoral pacemaker implant: It isn't what it seems! *PACE* 2004; **27**: 361–364.

32 Crossly GH, Gayle DD, Bailey JR et al. Defibrillator twiddler's syndrome causing device failure in a subpectoral transvenous system. *PACE* 1996; **19**: 376–377.

33 Wilkoff BL, Shimokochi DD, Schaal SF. Pacing rate increase due to application of steady external pressure on an activity-sensing pacemaker (Abstract). *PACE* 1987; **10**: 423.

34 Horenstein MS, Karpawich PP. Chronic performance of steroid-eluting epicardial leads in a growing pediatric population: a 10-year comparison. *PACE* 2003; **26**: 1467–1471.

35 Walker F, Siu SC, Woods S et al. Long-term outcomes of cardiac pacing in adults with congenital heart disease. *J Am Coll Cardiol* 2004; **43**: 1894–1901.

36 Karpawich PP, Hakami M, Arciniegas et al. Improved chronic epicardial pacing in children: Steroid contribution to porous platinized electrodes. *PACE* 1992; **15**: 1151–1157.

37 Karpawich P, Walters H, Hakimi M. Chronic performance of a transvenous steroid pacing lead used as an epi-intramyocardial electrode. *PACE* 1998; **21**: 1486–1488.

38 Hayes DL, Vlietstra RE Puga FJ et al. A novel approach to atrial endocardial pacing. *PACE* 1989; **12**: 125–130.

39 Juneja R, Saxena A, Choudhary S et al. Transatrial permanent pacing lead implantation in a patient of Ebstein's anomaly after one and half repair. *Indian Heart J* 2004; **56**: 670–672.

40 Byrd CL, Schwartz SJ. Transatrial implantation of transvenous pacing leads as an alternative to implantation of epicardial leads. *PACE* 1990; **13**: 1856–1859.

41 Westerman GR, Van Devanter SH. Transthoracic trans-atrial endocardial lead placement for permanent pacing. *Ann Thorac Surg* 1987; **43**: 445–446.

42 Karpawich PP. Chronic right ventricular pacing and cardiac performance: The pediatric perspective. *PACE* 2004; **27**: 844–849.

43 Karpawich PP, Justice CD, Cavitt DL et al. Developmental sequelae of fixed-rate ventricular pacing in the immature canine heart: An electrophysiologic, hemodynamic and histopathologic evaluation. *Am Heart J* 1991; **121**: 827–833.

44 Tantengco MV, Thomas RL, Karpawich PP. Left ventricular dysfunction following chronic right ventricular apical pacing in young patients. *J Am Coll Cardiol* 2001; **37**: 2093–2100.

45 Thambo JB, Bordachar P, Garrigue S et al. Detrimental ventricular remodelling in patients with congenital complete heart block and chronic right ventricular apical pacing. *Circulation* 2004; **110**: 3766–3772.

46 Sweeney MO, Hellkamp AS, Ellenbogen KA et al. Adverse effect of ventricular pacing on heart failure and atrial fibrillation among patients with normal baseline QRS duration in a clinical trial of pacemaker therapy for sinus node dysfunction. *Circulation* 2003; **107**: 2932–2937.

47 Mond HG, Gammage MD. Selective site pacing: The future of cardiac pacing? *PACE* 2004; **27**: 835–836.

48 Karpawich PP, Gates J, Stokes K. Septal His-Purkinje ventricular pacing in canines: A new endocardial electrode approach. *PACE* 1992; **15**: 2011–2015.

49 Deshmukh P, Romanyshyn M. Direct His-bundle pacing: Present and future. *PACE* 2004; **27**: 862–887.

50 Giudici MC, Karpawich PP. Alternative site pacing: It's time to define terms. *PACE* 1999; **22**: 551–553.

51 Karpawich PP, Mital S. Comparative left ventricular function following atrial, septal and apical single chamber right heart pacing in the young. *PACE* 1997; **20**: 1983–1988.

52 Lieberman R, Grenz D, Mond H et al. Selective site pacing: Defining and reaching the selected site. *PACE* 2004; **27**: 883–886.

53 Karpawich PP, Horenstein MS, Webster P. Site-specific right ventricular implant pacing to optimize paced left ventricular function in the young with and without congenital heart (Abstract). *PACE* 2002; **25**: 566.

54 Riedlbauchova L, Kautzner J, Hatala R et al. Is right ventricular outflow tract pacing an alternative to left ventricular/biventricular pacing? *PACE* 2004; **27**: 871–877.

55 Mond HG, Stokes KB. The electrode-tissue interface: The revolutionary role of steroid elution. *PACE* 1992; **15**: 95–107.

56 Hua W, Mond HG, Strathmore N. Chronic steroid-eluting lead performance: A comparison of atrial and ventricular pacing. *PACE* 1997; **20**: 17–24.

57 Mond HG, Hua W, Wang CC. Atrial pacing leads: The clinical contribution of steroid elution. *PACE* 1995; **18**: 1601–1608.

58 Hua W, Mond HG, Sparks P. The clinical performance of three designs of atrial pacing leads from a single manufacturer: The value of steroid elution. *Eur JCPE* 1996; **6**: 99–103.

59 Hidden-Lucet F, Halimi F, Gallais Y et al. Low chronic pacing thresholds of steroid-eluting active-fixation ventricular pacemaker leads: A useful alternative to passive-fixation leads. *PACE* 2000; **23**: 1978–1800.

60 Kistler PM, Liew G, Mond HG. Long-term performance of active-fixation pacing leads: A prospective study *PACE* 2006; **29**: 226–230.

61 Crossley G, Reynolds D, Brinkler JA et al. Permanent ventricular pacing from the right ventricular outflow tract or septum with an active fixation lead provides for excellent long term results (Abstract). *PACE* 1997; **20**: 1210.

62 Ward DE, Clarke B, Schofield PM et al. Long term transvenous ventricular pacing in adults with congenital abnormalities of the heart and great arteries. *Br Heart J* 1983; **50**: 325–329.

63 Hansky B, Blanz U, Peuster M et al. Endocardial pacing after Fontan-type procedures. *PACE* 2005; **28**: 140–148.

64 Chintala K, Forbes T, Karpawich PP. Effectiveness of transvenous pacemaker leads placed through intravascular stents in patients with congenital heart disease. *Am J Cardiol* 2005; **95**: 424–427.

65 Kistler PM, Sanders P, Davidson NC et al. The challenge of endocardial right ventricular pacing in patients with a tricuspid annuloplasty ring and severe tricuspid regurgitation. *PACE* 2002; **25**: 201–205.

66 Byrd C, Wilkoff B. Techniques and devices for extraction of pacemaker and implantable cardioverter-defibrillator leads. In: Ellenbogen K, Kay G, Wilkoff, eds. *Clinical Cardiac Pacing and Defibrillation.* WB Saunders, Philadelphia, PA, 2000: 695–709.

67 Mond Harry G. *The Cardiac Pacemaker. Function and Malfunction.* Harcourt Brace Jovanovich, New York 1983: 206.

68 Bai Y, Strathmore N, Mond H et al. Permanent ventricular pacing via the great cardiac vein. *PACE* 1994; **17**: 678–683.

69 Faerestrand S, Ohm Ole-Jørgen. Alternate pacing sites for patients with tricuspid valve prosthesis. *PACE* 2002; **25**: 234–238.

70 Curnis A, Mascioli G, Bianchetti F et al. Implantation of a single chamber pacemaker in patients with triple mechanical valve prosthesis: Utilization of coronary sinus distal branches to stimulate the left ventricle. *PACE* 2002; **25**: 239–240.

71 Garrigue S, Barold SS, Hocini M et al. Transvenous left atrial and left ventricular pacing in Ebstein's anomaly with severe interatrial conduction block. *PACE* 2001; **24**: 1032–1035.

72 Nguyen LS, Swaroop S, Prejean CA. Pacing in the middle cardiac vein in a patient with tricuspid prosthesis. *PACE* 2002; **25**: 243–244.

73 Bos HS, Pop GAM, Stel EA et al. Dual site coronary sinus pacing in a patient with an artificial tricuspid valve prosthesis. *PACE* 2004; **27**: 1451–1452.

74 Lucas R, Krabill K. Abnormal systemic venous connections. In: Emmanouilides et al., ed. *Heart Disease in Infants, Children and Adolescents*, 5th edn. Baltimore, Williams & Wilkins, 1995: 874–902.

75 Van Gelder BM, Elders J Bracke FA et al. Implantation of a biventricular pacing system in a patient with a coronary sinus not communicating with the right atrium. *PACE* 2003; **26**: 1294–1296

76 Tada H, Ito S, Naito S et al. Longitudinally partitioned coronary sinus: An unusual anomaly of the coronary venous system. *PACE* 2005; **28**: 352–353.

77 Kantoch MJ, McKay R, Tyrrell MJ. Left ventricular transvenous electrode dislodgement after Mustard repair for transposition of the great arteries. *PACE* 1993; **16**: 1887–1891.

78 Morquio L. Sur une maladie infantile et familiale caracterisee par des modifications permanentes du pouls des attaques syncopale et epileptiformes et la morte subite. *Arch Med Enf* 1901; **4**: 467–474.

79 Lev Maurice. Pathogenesis of congenital atrioventricular block. *Prog Cardiovasc Dis* 1972; **15**: 145–157.

80 Benson DW, Wang DW, Dyment M et al. Congenital sick sinus syndrome caused by recessive mutations in the cardiac sodium channel gene (SCN5A). *J Clin Invest* 2003; **112**: 1019–1028.

81 Schott JJ, Alshinawi C, Kyndt F, et al. Cardiac conduction defects associated with mutations in SCN5A. *Nat Genet* 1999; **23**: 201–221.

82 Groenewegen WA, Firouzi M, Bezzina CR et al. A cardiac sodium channel mutation cosegregates with a rare connexin 40 genotype in familial atrial standstill. *Circ Res* 2002; 92: 14–22.

83 Kurita T, Ohe T, Marui N et al. Bradycardia-induced abnormal QT prolongation in patients with complete atrioventricular block with torsade de pointes. *Am J Cardiol* 1992; **69**: 628–633.

84 Anderson RH, Wenick ACG, Losekoot TG et al. Congenitally complete heart block. Developmental aspects. *Circulation* 1977; **56**: 90–101.

85 Bharati S, McCue CM, Tingelstad JB et al. Lack of connection between the atria and the peripheral conduction system in a case of corrected transposition with congenital atrioventricular block. *Am J Cardiol* 1978; **42**: 147–153.

86 Gerlis LM, Anderson RH, Becker AE. Complete heart block as a consequence of atrionodal discontinuity. *Br Heart J* 1975; **37**: 345–356.

87 Lev M, Cuadros H, Paul MH. Interruption of the atrioventricular bundle with congenital atrioventricular block. *Circulation* 1971; **43**: 703–710.

88 Bharati S, Lev M. Congenital abnormalities of the conducting system in sudden death in young adults. *J Am Coll Cardiol* 1986; **8**: 1096–1104.

89 Husson GS, Blackman MS, Rogers MC et al. Familial congenital bundle branch system disease. *Am J Cardiol* 1973; **32**: 365–369.

90 Rosen KM, Mehta A, Rahimtoola SH et al. Sites of congenital and surgical heart block as defined by His bundle electrocardiography. *Circulation* 1971; **44**: 833–841.

91 Kelly DT, Brodsky SJ, Mirowski M et al. Bundle of His recordings in congenital complete heart block. *Circulation* 1972; **45**: 277–280.

92 Nasrallah AT, Gillette PC, Mullins CE. Congenital and surgical atrioventricular block within the His bundle. *Am J Cardiol* 1975; **36**: 914–920.

93 James TN, Spencer MS, Kloepfer JC. De Subitaneis Mortibus. XXI. Adult onset syncope, with comments on the nature of congenital heart block and the morphogenesis of the human atrioventricular septal junction. *Circulation* 1976; **54**: 1001–1009.

94 Sarachek NS, Leonard JJ. Familial heart block and sinus bradycardia. Classification and natural history. *Am J Cardiol* 1972; **29**: 451–458.

95 Stephan E. Hereditary bundle branch system defect. *Am Heart J* 1978; **95**: 89–95.

96 Morgans CM, Gray KE, Robb GH. A survey of familial heart block. *Br Heart J* 1974; **36**: 693–696.

97 Lynch HT, Mohiuddin S, Moran J et al. Hereditary progressive atrioventricular conduction defect. *Am J Cardiol* 1975; **36**: 297–301.

98 Greenspahn BR, Denes P, Daniel W et al. Chronic bifascicular block: Evaluation of familial factors. *Ann Intern Med* 1976; **84**: 521–525.

99 Graber HL, Unverferth DV, Baker PB et al. Evolution of a hereditary cardiac conduction and muscle disorder: A study involving a family with six generations affected. *Circulation* 1986; **74**: 21–35.

100 Tucker KJ, Murphy J, Conti JB et al. Syncope and sinus arrest associated with the upper limb-cardiovascular (Holt-Oram) syndrome. *PACE* 1994; **17**: 1678–1680.

101 Silverman ME, Copeland AJ, Hurst JW. The Holt-Oram syndrome: The long and the short of it. *Am J Cardiol* 1970; **25**: 11–17.

102 Kearns TP, Sayre GP. Retinitis pigmentosa, external ophthalmoplegia and complete heart block. *Arch Ophthalmol* 1958; **60**: 280–289.

103 Charles R, Holt S, Kay JM et al. Myocardial ultrastructure and the development of atrioventricular block in Kearns-Sayre syndrome. *Circulation* 1981; **63**: 214–219.

104 Young TJ, Shah AK, Lee MH et al. Kearns-Sayre syndrome: A case report and review of cardiovascular complications. *PACE* 2005; **28**: 454–457.

105 Ulicny KS, Detterbeck FC, Hall CD. Sinus dysrhythmia in Kearns-Sayre syndrome. *PACE* 1994; **17**: 991–994.

106 Ross BA. Congenital complete atrioventricular block. *Pediatr Clin North Am* 1990; **37**: 69–78.

107 Lee LA, Coulter S, Erner S et al. Cardiac immunoglobulin deposition in congenital heart block associated with maternal anti-Ro autoantibodies. *Am J Med* 1987; **83**: 793–796.

108 Taylor PV, Scott JS, Gerlis LM et al. Maternal antibodies against fetal cardiac antigens in congenital complete heart block. *N Engl J Med* 1986; **315**: 667–672.

109 Goble MM, Dick M II, McCune et al. Atrioventricular conduction in children of women with systemic lupus erythematosus. *Am J Cardiol* 1993; **71**: 94–98.

110 Schmidt KG, Ulmer HE, Silverman NH et al. Perinatal outcome of fetal complete atrioventricular block: A multicenter experience. *J Am Coll Cardiol* 1991; **17**: 1360–1366.

111 Smeenk RJT. Immunological aspects of congenital atrioventricular block. *PACE* 1007; **20**: 2093–2097.

112 O'Connor BK, Gillette P. Congenital heart block: Natural history and management. *ACC Current J Rev* 1995; **Mar/Apr**: 63–65.

113 Buyon J, Roubey R, Swersky S et al. Complete congenital heart block: Risk of occurrence and therapeutic approach to prevention. *J Rheumatol* 1988; **15**: 1104–1105.

114 Lewman LV, Demany MA, Zimmerman HA. Congenital tumor of atrioventricular node with complete heart block and sudden death. *Am J Cardiol* 1972; **29**: 554–557.

115 Moak J, Barron KS, Hougen TJ et al. Congenital heart block: Development of late-onset cardiomyopathy, a previously underappreciated sequela. *J Am Coll Cardiol* 2001; **37**: 238–242.

116 Thery CL, Lekieffre J, Dupuis CL. Atrioventricular block secondary to a congenital aneurysm of the membranous septum. Histological examination of conduction system. *Br Heart J* 1975; **37**: 1097–1100.

117 Esscher EB. Congenital complete heart block in adolescence and adult life. A follow-up study. *Eur Heart J* 1981; **2**: 281–288.

118 Karpawich PP, Gillette PC, Garson A et al. Congenital complete atrioventricular block: Clinical and electrophysiologic predictors of need for pacemaker insertion. *Am J Cardiol* 1981; **48**: 1098–1102.

119 Winkler RB, Freed MD, Nadas AS. Exercise-induced ventricular ectopy in children and young adults with complete heart block. *Am Heart J* 1980; **99**: 87–92.

120 Molthan ME, Miller RA, Hastreiter AR et al. Congenital heart block with fatal Adams-Stokes attacks in childhood. *Pediatrics* 1962; **30**: 32–35.

121 Michaelsson M, Jonzon A, Riesenfeld T. Isolated congenital complete atrioventricular block in adult life: A prospective study. *Circulation* 1995; **92**: 442–449.

122 Michaelsson M, Riesenfeld T, Jonzon A. Natural history of congenital complete atrioventricular block. *PACE* 1997; **20**: 2098–2101.

123 Walsh CA, McAlister HF, Andrews CA et al. Pacemaker implantation in children: A 21-year experience. *PACE* 1988; **11**: 1940–1944.

124 Campbell M, Emanuel R. Six cases of congenital heart block followed for 30–40 years. *Br Heart J* 1967; **29**: 577–587.

125 Corne RA, Mathewson AL. Congenital complete atrioventricular block. *Am J Cardiol* 1972: 29: 12–421.

126 Bharati S, Lev M. Congenital abnormalities of the conduction system in sudden death in young adults. *J Am Coll Cardiol* 1986; **8**: 1096–1104.

127 Ngarmukos T, Werres R. Normal sinus rhythm in a patient with corrected transposition of great arteries after 30 years of complete heart block. *PACE* 1999; **22**: 1116–1117.

128 Strieper M. Karpawich P, Frias P et al. Initial experience with cardiac resynchronization therapy in young patients with ventricular dysfunction and congenital heart disease. *Am J Cardiol* 2004; **94**: 1352–1354.

129 Dubin A, Cecchin F, Law, I et al. Resynchronization therapy in pediatric and congenital heart disease patients: A multicenter study. *Heart Rhythm* (Abstract) 2004; **1**: S50.

130 Horenstein MS, Karpawich PP. Pacemaker syndrome in the young: Do children need dual chamber as the initial pacing mode? *PACE* 2004; **27**: 600–605.

131 Friedman RA, Fenrich AL, Kertesz NJ. Congenital complete atrioventricular block. *PACE* 2001; **24**: 1681–1688.

132 Griffiths SP. Congenital complete heart block (Editorial). *Circulation* 1971; **43**: 615–617.

133 Bharati S, McCue CM, Tingelstad JB et al. Lack of connection between the atria and the peripheral conduction system in a case of corrected transposition with congenital atrioventricular block. *Am J Cardiol* 1978; **42**: 147–153.

134 Daliento L, Corrado D, Buja G et al. Rhythm and conduction disturbances in isolated congenitally corrected transposition of the great arteries. *Am J Cardiol* 1986; **58**: 314–318.

135 Lundstrom U, Bull C, Wyse RKH et al. The natural and "unnatural" history of congenitally corrected transposition. *Am J Cardiol* 1990; **65**: 1222–1229.

136 Yeşil M, Bayata S, Postaci N et al. New onset complete heart block and corrected transposition of great arteries in the seventh decade. *PACE* 1997; **20**: 134–135.

137 Amikan S, Lemar J, Kishon Y et al. Complete heart block in an adult with corrected transposition of the great arteries treated with a permanent pacemaker. *Thorax* 1979; **34**: 547–549.

138 Estes NAM, Salem DN, Isner JM et al. Permanent pacemaker therapy in corrected transposition of the great arteries: Analysis of site of lead placement in 40 patients. *Am J Cardiol* 1983; **52**: 1091–1097.

139 Medina-Ravell V, Castellanos A, Portillo-Agosta B et al. Management of tachyarrhythmias with dual-chamber pacemakers. *PACE* 1983; **6**: 333–345.

140 Roy PR, Emanuel R, Ismail SA et al. Hereditary prolongation of the Q-T interval: Genetic observations and management in three families with twelve affected members. *Am J Cardiol* 1976; **37**: 237–243.

141 Di Segni E, David D, Katzenstein M et al. Permanent overdrive pacing for the suppression of recurrent ventricular tachycardia in a newborn with long QT syndrome. *J Electrocardiol* 1980; **13**: 189–192.

142 Eldar M, Griffin, Abbott JA et al. Permanent cardiac pacing in patients with the long QT syndrome. *J Am Coll Cardiol* 1987; **10**: 600–607.

143 Han J, Moe GK. Nonuniform recovery of excitability in ventricular muscle. *Circ Res* 1964; **14**: 44–60.

144 Singer DH, Lazzara R, Hoffman. Interrelationships between automaticity and conduction in Purkinje fibers. *Circ Res* 1967; **21**: 537–558.

145 Schechter E, Freeman CC, Lazzara R. Afterpotentials as a mechanism for the long QT syndrome: Electrophysiologic studies of a case. *J Am Coll Cardiol* 1984; **3**: 1556–1561.

146 Sharma S, Nair KG, Gadekar HA. Romano-Ward prolonged QY syndrome with intermittent T wave alternans and atrioventricular block. *Am Heart J* 1981; **101**: 500–501.

147 Bharati S, Dreifus L, Bucheleres G et al. The conduction system in patients with a prolonged QT interval. *J Am Coll Cardiol* 1985; **6**: 1110–1109.

148 Hagen PT, Scholz DG, Edwards WD. Incidence and size of patent foramen ovale during the first ten decades of life. An autopsy study of 965 normal hearts. *Mayo Clin Proc* 1984; **59**: 17–21.

149 Emmanuel R, O'brien K, Somerville J et al. Association of secundum atrial septal defect with abnormalities of atrioventricular conduction or left axis deviation. Genetic study of 10 families. *Br Heart J* 1975; **37**: 1085–1092.

150 Pease WE, Nordenberg A, Ladda RL. Familial atrial septal defect with prolonged atrioventricular conduction. *Circulation* 1976; **53**: 759–762.

151 Bizzaro RO, Callahan JA Feldt RH et al. Familial atrial septal defect with prolonged atrioventricular conduction. *Circulation* 1970; **41**: 677–679.

152 Kahler RL, Braunwald E, Plauth WH et al. Familial congenital heart disease: Familial occurrence of atrial septal defect with A-V conduction abnormalities; supravalvular aortic and pulmonic stenosis: and ventricular septal defect. *Am J Med* 1966; **40**: 384–387.

153 Björnstad PG. Secundum type atrial septal defect with prolonged P-R interval and autosomal dominant mode of inheritance. *Br Heart J* 1974; **1974**: 1149–1153.

154 Karpawich PP, Antillon JR, Cappola PR et al. Pre- and postoperative electro-physiologic assessment of children with secundum atrial septal defect. *Am J Cardiol* 1985; **55**: 519–521.

155 Van Erckelens F, Sigmund M, Lambertz H et al. Asymptomatic left ventricular malposition of a transvenous pacemaker lead through a sinus venosus defect: Follow-up over 17 years. *PACE* 1991; **14**: 989–993.

156 Sharifi M, Sorkin R, Lakier JB. Left heart pacing and cardioembolic stroke. *PACE* 1994; **17**: 1691–1696.

157 Ross WB, Mohiuddin SM, Pagano T et al. Malposition of a transvenous cardiac electrode associated with amaurosis fugax. *PACE* 1983; **6**: 119–124.

158 Tobin AM, Grodman RS, Fisherkeller M et al. Two-dimensional echocardiographic localization of a malpositioned pacing catheter. *PACE* 1983; **6**: 291–299.

159 Schiavone WA, Castle L, Salcedo E et al. Amaurosis Fugax in a patient with a left ventricular endocardial pacemaker. *PACE* 1984; **7**: 288–292.

160 Flicker S, Eldredge WJ, Naidech HJ et al. Computed tomographic localiza-tion of malposition of pacing electrodes: The value of cardiovascular computed tomography. *PACE* 1985; **8**: 589–599.

161 Shmuely H, Erdman S, Strasberg B et al. Seven years of left ventricular pacing due to malposition of pacing electrode. *PACE* 1992; **15**: 369–372.

162 Splittgerber FH, Ulbricht LJ, Reifschneider HJ et al. Left ventricular malposition of a transvenous cardioverter defibrillator lead: A case report. *PACE* 1993; **16**: 1066–1069.

163 Zilberman M, Karpawich PP. Alternate Site Atrial Pacing in the Young: Echocardi-ographic indices of atrial function (Abstract). *Circulation* 2005; **112**: II-734.

164 Steinberg I, Dubilier W, Lukas D. Persistence of left superior vena cava. *Dis Chest* 1953; **24**: 479–484.

165 Mantini E, Grondin C, Lillehei W et al. Congenital abnormalities involving the coronary sinus. *Circulation* 1966; **33**: 317–324.

166 Lenox CC, Zuberbuhler JR, Park SC et al. Absent right superior vena cava with persistent left superior vena cava: Implications and management. *Am J Cardiol* 1980; **45**: 117–122.

167 Camm AJ, Dymond D, Spurrell AJ. Sinus node dysfunction associated with absence of right superior vena cava. *Br Heart J* 1979; **41**: 504–517.

168 Lenox CC, Hashida Y, Anderson RH et al. Conduction tissue abnormalities in absence of the right superior caval vein. *Int J Cardiol.* 1985; **8**: 251–254.

169 Harthorne JW, Dinsmore RE, Desanctis RW. Superior vena caval anomaly prevent-ing pervenous pacemaker implantation. *Br Heart J* 1969; **31**: 809–812.

170 Garcia L, Levine RS, Kossowsky W et al. Persistent left superior vena cava complicating pacemaker catheter insertion. *Chest* 1972; **61**: 396–399.

171 Kukral JC. Transvenous pacemaker failure due to anomalous venous return to the heart. *Chest* 1971; **59**: 458–460.

172 Dirix LY, Kersschot IE, Fierens H et al. Implantation of a dual chamber pacemaker in a patient with persistent left superior vena cava. *PACE* 1988; **11**: 343–345.

173 Rønnevik PK, Abrahamsen AM, Tollefsen I. Transvenous pacemaker implantation via a unilateral left superior vena cava. *PACE* 1982; **5**: 808–813.

174 Ashida Y, Mori T, Kuroda H et al. Transvenous dual chamber pacing via a unilateral left superior vena cava. *PACE* 1998; **21**: 137–139.

175 Antonelli D, Rosenfeld T. Implantation of dual chamber pacemaker in a patient with persistent left superior vena cava. *PACE* 1997; **20**: 1737–1738.

176 Hellestrand KJ, Ward DE, Bexton RS et al. The use of active fixation electrodes for permanent endocardial pacing via a left superior vena cava. *PACE* 1982; **5**: 180–184.

177 Okreglicki AM, Scott Millar RN. VDD pacing in persistent left superior vena cava. *PACE* 1998; **21**: 1189–1191.

178 Mattke S, Markewitz A, Dorwarth U et al. Defibrillator implantation via persistent left superior vena cava. *PACE* 1995; **18**: 117–120.

179 Brooks R, Jackson G, McGovern B et al. Transvenous cardioverter-defibrillator implantation via persistent left superior vena cava. *Am Heart J* 1995; **129**: 195–197.

180 Paulussen GMG, Van Gelder BM. Implantation of a biventricular pacing system in a patient with a persistent left superior vena cava. *PACE* 2004; **27**: 1014–1016.

181 Lyon X, Kappenberger L. Implantation of a cardiac resynchronization system for idiopathic dilated cardiomyopathy in a patient with persistent left superior vena cava using an experimental lead for left ventricular stimulation. *PACE* 2000; **23**: 1439–1441.

182 Ng KS, Foo D, Lim J. His-bundle pacing in a patient with persistent left superior vena cava. *PACE* 2005; **28**: 588–590.

183 Chaithiraphan S, Goldberg E, Wolff W et al. Massive thrombosis of the coronary sinus as an unusual complication of transvenous pacemaker insertion in a patient with persistent left, and no right superior vena cava. *J Am Geriatric Soc* 1974; **22**: 79–85.

184 Villani GQ, Piepoli M, Quaretti P et al. Cardiac pacing in unilateral left superior vena cava: Evaluation by digital angiography. *PACE* 1991; **14**: 1566–1567.

185 Birnie D, Tang ASL. Permanent pacing from a left ventricular vein in a patient with persistent left and absent right superior vena cava. *PACE* 2000; **23**: 2135–2137.

186 Dosios T, Gorgogiannis, G, Sakorafas G et al. Persistent left superior vena cava: A problem in the transvenous pacing of the heart. *PACE* 1991; **14**: 389–390.

187 Hussain SA, Chakravarty SA, Chaikhouni A et al. Congenital absence of superior vena cava: Unusual anomaly of superior systemic veins complicating pacemaker implantation. *PACE* 1981; **4**: 328–334.

188 Robbens EJ, Ruiter JH. Atrial pacing via unilateral persistent left superior vena cava. *PACE* 1986; **9**: 594–596.

189 Van Mierop LHS, Kutscher LM, Victorica BE. Ebstein's Anomaly. In: Adams FH, Emmanouilides GC, Riemenschneider TA, eds. *Moss' Heart Disease in Infants, Children and Adolescents*, 4th edn. Williams & Wilkins, Baltimore, USA, 1989: 361–371.

190 Netter FH. *Heart*: The Ciba collection of medical illustrations. Ciba Geigy Corporation. 1978: 143–144.

191 Anderson KR, Zuberbuhler JR, Anderson RH et al. True spectrum of Ebstein's Anomaly of the heart: A review. *Mayo Clin Proc* 1979; **54**: 174–180.

192 Till J, Celermajer D, Deanfield J. The natural history of arrhythmias in Ebstein's anomaly (Abstract). *J Am Coll Cardiol* 1992; **19**(3): 293-A.

193 Kumar AE, Fyler DC, Meittinen OS et al. Ebstein's anomaly. Clinical profile and natural history. *Am J Cardiol* 1971; **28**: 84–95.

194 Allen MR, Hayes DL, Warnes CA et al. Permanent pacing in Ebstein's anomaly. *PACE* 1997; **20**: 1243–1246.

195 Pierard LA, Fenrard L, Demoulin JC. Persistent atrial standstill in familial Ebstein's anomaly. *Br Heart J* 1985; **53**: 594–597.

196 Price JE, Amsterdam EA, Vera Z. Ebstein's disease associated with complete atrio ventricular block. *Chest* 1978; **73**: 542–544.

197 Rothfield EL, Zucker IR, Kannerstein M. Stokes Adams syndrome and Ebstein's anomaly. *Angiology* 1973; **24**: 332–337.

198 Ng R, Sommerville J, Ross D. Ebstein's anomaly: Late results of surgical correction. *Eur J Cardiol* 1979; **9**: 39–52.

199 Fujiwara T, Kawada M, Harada M et al. Successful case of tricuspid valve replacement His bundle interruption and atrioventricular sequential pacemaker implantation for Ebstein's anomaly with Wolff-Parkinson-White syndrome. *J Jpn Assoc Thorac Surg* 1984; **32**: 82–87.

200 Jayaprakash S, Mond HG, Sparks PB et al. Transvenous ventricular pacing options in Ebstein's anomaly. *Indian Heart J* 1998; **50**: 565–568.

201 Andersen C, Oxhøj H, Justensen P. Pacing in a patient with Ebstein's anomaly. *PACE* 1989; **12**: 1586–1588.

202 Mustard WT, Keith JD, Trusler GA et al. The surgical management of transposition of the great vessels. *J Thorac Cardiovasc Surg* 1964; **48**: 953–958.

203 Mustard WT. Successful two stage correction of transposition of the great vessels. *Surgery* 1964; **55**: 469–472.

204 Wilson NJ, Clarkson PM, Barratt-Boyes BG et al. Long-term outcome after the Mustard repair for simple transposition of the great arteries: 28-year follow-up. *J Am Coll Cardiol* 1998; **32**: 758–765.

205 Hayes CJ, Gersony WM. Arrhythmias after the Mustard operation for transposition of the great arteries: A long-term study. *J Am Coll Cardiol* 1986; **7**: 133–137.

206 Bink-Boelkens MTh E, Velvis H, Homan van der Heide JJ et al. Dysrhythmias after atrial surgery in children. *Am Heart J* 1983; **106**: 125–130.

207 Williams W, Goldman B, Irwin M et al. Permanent cardiac pacing after Mustard's operation for repair of transposition (Abstract). *PACE* 1989; **12**: 679.

208 Hesslein PS, Gutgesell HP, Gillette PC et al. Exercise assessment of sinoatrial node function following the Mustard operation. *Am Heart J* 1982; **103**: 351–356.

209 Gillette PC, Kugler JD, Garson A et al. Mechanisms of cardiac arrhythmias after the Mustard operation for transposition of the great arteries. *Am J Cardiol* 1980; **45**: 1225–1230.

210 Trusler GA, Williams WG, Duncan KF et al. Results with the Mustard operation in simple transposition of the great arteries. *Ann Surg* 1987; **206**: 251–260.

211 Takahashi M, Lindesmith GG, Lewis AB et al. Long-term results of the Mustard procedure. *Circulation* 1977; **56**: ii-85–90.

212 Clarkson PM, Barratt-Boyes BG, Neutze JM. Late dysrhythmias and disturbances of conduction following Mustard operation for complete transposition of the great arteries. *Circulation* 1976; **53**: 519–524.

213 Kammeraad JAE, van Deurzen CHM, Sreeram N et al. Predictors of sudden cardiac death after Mustard or Senning repair for transposition of the great arteries. *J Am Coll Cardiol* 2004; **44**: 1095–1102.

214 Senning A. Surgical correction of transposition of the great vessels. *Surgery* 1959; **45**: 966–977.

215 Bender HW, Graham TP, Boucek RJ et al. Comparative operative results of the Senning and Mustard procedures for transposition of the great arteries. *Circulation* 1980; **62**: 197–203.

216 Quaegebeur JM, Rohmer J, Brom AG et al. Revival of the Senning operation for treatment of transposition of the great arteries. *Thorax* 1977; **32**: 517–524.

217 Deanfield J, Camm J, Macartney F et al. Arrhythmia and late mortality after Mustard and Senning operation for transposition of the great arteries. *J Thorac Cardiovasc Surg* 1988; **96**: 569–576.

218 Jatene AD, Fontes VF, Souza LC et al. Anatomic correction of transposition of the great arteries. *J Thorac Cardiovasc Surg* 1982; **83**: 20–26.

219 Mond H, Kertes P, Hunt D et al. Permanent pacing in children having transposition of the great vessels corrected by the Mustard procedure (Abstract). *PACE* 1984; **7**: 473.

220 Gillette PC, Wampler DG, Shannon C et al. Use of cardiac pacing after the Mustard operation for transposition of the great arteries. *J Am Coll Cardiol* 1986; **7**: 138–141.

221 Knauf DG, Selby JH, Alexander JA. Left atrial pacing following Mustard's correction of transposition of the great vessels. *Chest* 1982; **81**: 374–376.

222 Turley K, Hanley FL, Verrier ED et al. The Mustard procedure in infant (less than 100 days of age). Ten year follow-up. *J Thorac Cardiovasc Surg* 1988; **96**: 849–853.

223 Gillette PC, Shannon C, Blair H et al. Transvenous pacing in pediatric patients. *Am Heart J* 1983; **105**: 843–847.

224 Handler CE, Walker JM. Permanent transvenous pacing after a Mustard procedure. *PACE* 1990; **13**: 2100–2103.

225 Krongrad, E, Bharati S, Sternfeld L et al. Histolic observations of the cardiac conducting system in a heart with post operative bilateral bundle branch block. *Am J Cardiol* 1977; **40**: 635–641.

226 Titus JL, Daugherty GW, Kirklin JW. Lesions of the atrioventricular conduction system after repair of ventricular septal defect: Relation to heart block. *Circulation* 1963; **28**: 82–87.

227 Pahlajani DB, Serratto M, Mehta A et al. Surgical bifascicular block. *Circulation* 1975; **52**: 82–87.

228 Murphy DA, Tynan M, Graham GR et al. Prognosis of complete atrioventricular dissociation in children after open-heart surgery. *The Lancet* 1970: 750–752.

229 Cairns JA, Dobell ARC, Gibbons JE et al. Prognosis of right bundle branch block and left anterior hemiblock after intracardiac repair of tetralogy of Fallot. *Am Heart J* 1975; **90**: 549–554.

230 Moss AJ, Klyman G, Emmanouilides GC. Late onset complete heart block. Newly recognised sequela of cardiac surgery. *Am J Cardiol* 1972; **30**: 884–887.

231 Karpawich PP, Jackson WL, Cavitt DL et al. Late onset unprecedented complete atrioventricular block following tetralogy of Fallot repair: Electrophysiologic findings. *Am Heart J* 1987; **114**: 654–656.

232 Sondheimer HM, Izukawa T, Olley PM et al. Conduction disturbances after total correction of tetralogy of Fallot. *Am Heart J* 1976; **92**: 278–28; *PACE* 1997; **20**: 17–24. 2.

233 Quattlebaum TG, Varghese PJ, Neill CA et al. Sudden death among postoperative patients with tetralogy of Fallot. A follow-up study of 243 patients for an average of twelve years. *Circulation* 1976; **54**: 289–293.

234 Bink-Boelkens MTh E, Velvis H, Homan van der Heide JJ et al. Dysrhythmias after atrial surgery in children. *Am Heart J* 1983; **106**: 125–130.

235 Fallot A. Contribution a l'anatomie pathologique de la maladie bleue (cyanose cardiaque). *Marseillee Medical* 1888; **25**: 77.

236 Rao BNS, Anderson RC, Edwards JE. Anatomic variations in tetralogy of Fallot. *Am Heart J* 1971; **81**: 361–365.

237 Garson A, Porter C, Gillette P et al. Induction of ventricular tachycardia during electrophysiologic study after repair of tetralogy of Fallot. *J Am Coll Cardiol* 1983; **1**: 1493–1502.

238 Taliercio CP, McGoon MD, Vlietstra RE et al. Cardiac pacing after the Fontan procedure: 1973–1986. *Clin Prog Pacing and EP* 1986; **3**: 246–254.

239 Dilawar M, Bradley SM, Saul JP et al. Sinus node dysfunction after intraatrial lateral tunnel and extracardiac conduit Fontan procedures. *Paediatric Cardiol* 2003; **24**: 284–288.

240 Kaulitz R, Ziemer G, Paul T et al. Fontan-type procedures: Residual lesions and late interventions. *Ann Thorac Surg* 2002; **74**: 778–785.

241 Ward De, Clarke B, Schofield PM et al. Long term ventricular transvenous pacing in adults with congenital abnormalities of the heart and great arteries. *Br Heart J* 1983; **50**: 325–329.

242 Cohen MI, Wernovsky G, Vetter VL et al. Sinus node function after a systematically staged Fontan procedure. *Circulation* 1998; **98**: II 352–359.

243 Manning PB, Mayer JE, Wernovsky G et al. Staged operation to Fontan increases the incidence of sinoatrial dysfunction. *J Thorac Cardiovasc Surg* 1996; **111**: 833–834.

244 Shah MJ, Nehgme R, Carboni M et al. Endocardial atrial pacing lead implantation and midterm follow-up in young patients with sinus node dysfunction after the Fontan procedure. *PACE* 2004; **27**: 949–954.

245 Ramesh V, Gaynor JW, Shah MJ et al. Comparison of left and right atrial epicardial pacing in patients with congenital heart disease. *Ann Thorac Surg* 1999; **68**: 2314–2319.

246 Kucharzuk JC, Cohen MI, Rhodes LA. Epicardial atrial pacemaker lead placement after multiple cardiac operations. *Ann Thorac Surg* 2001; **71**: 2057–2058.

247 Cohen MI, Vetter VL, Bush DM et al. Epicardial pacemaker implantation and follow-up in patients with a single ventricle after the Fontan operation. *J Thorac Cardiovasc Surg* 2001; **121**: 804–811.

248 Johnsrude CK, Backer CL, Deal BJ et al. Transmural atrial pacing in patients with postoperative congenital heart disease. *J Cardiovasc Electrophysiol* 1999; **10**: 351–357.

249 Vince DJ, Tyers GFO, Kerr CR. Transvenous atrial pacing in the management of sick sinus syndrome following surgical treatment of the univentricular heart: Case report and review. *PACE* 1986; **9**: 441–448.

250 Warfield DA, Hayes D, VonFeldt LK et al. Permanent pacing in patients with univentricular heart (Abstract). *PACE* 1994; **17**: 806.

251 Blackburn MEC, Gibbs JL. Ventricular pacing from the coronary sinus in a patient with a Fontan circulation. *Br Heart J* 1993; **70**: 578–579.

252 Bens JL, Goudot B, Alsac J et al. Permanent endocardial pacing in a case of single ventricle submitted to Fontan's operation. *Stimucoeur* 1985; **13**: 271–275.

253 Adwani SS, Sreeram N, DeGiovanni JV. Percutaneous transhepatic dual chamber pacing in children with Fontan circulation. *Heart* 1997; **77**: 574–575.

254 West JNW, Shearmann CP, Gammage MD. Permanent pacemaker positioning via the inferior vena cava in a case of single ventricle with loss of right atrial-vena cava continuity. *PACE* 1993; **16**: 1753–1755.

255 Webb C, Jenkins K, Karpawich P, et al. Collaborative Care for Adults with Congenital Heart Disease. *Circulation* 2002; **105**: 2318–2323.

Index

Note: Page numbers in *italics* refer to figures and tables.